Totally Healthy

On Purpose

DR. TOM TUFTS

PASTOR VINNY KORB

KATE JUNEAU

DEB ST. CYR-PAUL

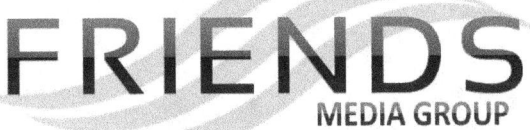

I0439332

Totally Healthy

On Purpose

Taking the necessary steps to 'get healthy,' in any area of life, requires several essential elements. With each component we discover an attitude, or perspective, that is also necessary in order to improve.

It is relatively easy to 'say' that we want to become healthy. It's an entirely different commitment to say, "I am going to do whatever it takes to become healthy" and *then follow through.* No matter the area of life, finances, spiritual healthy, physical health, relational or emotional health, *'if it's important, it's intentional'* has to become a reality.

Generally, we look for guidance that is specific to our intentions. If you wanted to learn how to play the piano, it would not be beneficial to take lessons *if the lessons were in karate.* In other words, we begin a journey with some sort of specific goal in mind. Stephen Covey calls it "beginning with the end in mind" in *The Seven Habits of Highly Successful People.*

We usually want this guidance and direction from people who have been trained in the field, or at the least, have experienced it themselves and accomplished the same goal that we have. Having a trained body-builder as a coach is probably not helpful if you are trying to learn ballet. That's why they have all of the different kind of doctors: They specialize in one area of expertise.

When we receive professional, expert advice, it requires a 'humble' heart and attitude to be able to accept their insights. As a former teaching professional (PGA Golf Professional) I can tell you that country clubs, airplanes, business meetings and driving ranges are full of people who *think they are experts.* In golf we used to say, "Women will take lessons and never practice. Men will practice and never take lessons." You can't improve at golf without both pieces: If the greatest golfers in the world have coaches and they are continually adjusting their swings, then what makes the rest of us think that we can improve on our own?

Acknowledging that the 'teacher' knows more than you do, that they are probably right, and that you need to adjust to their expertise, *requires a humble heart.* Right here, many people hit the wall of self-improvement. They are not open to other perspectives. They will not admit their own short-comings. *It's easier to remain sick, deformed, wounded and terminally ill than it is to change.*

Once there is an established path then it is up to us to put it into action. I have yet to discover anything that is any worthwhile significance, happened without effort and by accident. Getting healthy, in any way, takes hard work. It's mentally taxing. It's emotionally draining. It's physically demanding. It's spiritually challenging. It's financially expensive.

But the change is worth it.

The Bible says that mankind was 'created in the image of God.' I don't believe all the hype that you hear from pulpits across the country about how 'prosperous' (financially wealthy) we are supposed to be or that we will never have an illness or a need. But I do believe this: You were designed by God to be a healthy person, in healthy relationships enjoying all that life has to offer.

The question this book is focused on is simple: What is keeping you from that kind of life?

For me, usually the answer is also *me.*

In the counseling world, the old saying goes like this:

Until the pain of change is less than the pain of staying the same, nothing will change.

So imagine that on a scale of one to ten, the discomfort level in your life is a seven. And the thought of changing your lifestyle causes you such anguish that it seems like a nine. In this case, it's easier (more comfortable) to stay where we are, in spite of the discomfort, than to put ourselves through the pain of change.

But if our level of pain is at an eight, and we see the challenge of the adjustments as a seven, then it's *more comfortable to change than to remain the same.* **Until we view our opportunity this way, as a means to find more comfort, it's unlikely we will change much, if anything at all.**

In other words, until our painful, sick lives are less attractive than a healthy, vibrant, growing life, we will stay wounded, sick, injured and full of angst. That's not the life we were designed for. *That's not the life we dreamed of as children and that's not the life we want as adults.* **So why settle for it?**

You don't have to settle for it. But to obtain the reward, there is a price to pay. The price is to get your ego under control, submit to the experts experience and advice, and get your feet and life moving where your heart and mind want to be.

Before we get too far, let me put this on the table.

I'm not an expert on much of anything. In reality, I am not an expert on anything. I have done some things right, and done some things well, in some respects. But I am human and have made more than my share of glaring, ridiculous, foolish, immature mistakes. In fact, my failures exceed my successes by a mile.

There is one contest I am winning. My attempts outnumber my failures by *one. The key to success isn't to never fail; it's to never fail to try.* As my family says, "Even a blind hog finds an acorn once in a while." In the famous words of Dore' from *"Finding Nemo,"* Just keep swimming, just keep swimming. The ocean is huge, and life's adventure is bigger than that. There's so much you have yet to discover!

In order to help you I have enlisted the help of some experts on nutrition, cooking and counseling issues. These are men and women who really 'get it' and can help you. Give their words great value and weight. They have committed themselves to these issues in order to be able to help people along the way. You are one of those people!

Keep trying. Keep swimming. Keep on keeping on.

You can't see the White House unless you go to Washington, D.C. If that's where you want to end up, you have to start with your destination in mind. Sure, you can get there a million ways. You can get there by way of Australia, if you want to. *But the important piece of the puzzle is that you know when you have arrived at your destination.*

What's your purpose? When it's all said and done, what will you be remembered for? How will you know when your life's mission is complete?

If you don't know where you want to end up, you are not ready to get started moving forward.

Take the time to write this out: My life's purpose is:

Question: How will you accomplish this unless you are Totally Healthy?

Take time to write out an answer. [Usually, the answer is, "I can't."]

If it's important, it's intentional. I will live my life, Totally Healthy, On Purpose.

Signed: _____

Date _____

Totally Healthy

On Purpose

What Does It Mean To Be Spiritually Healthy?

A Spiritually Healthy Person Understands the Biblical Perspective of the Spiritual Condition of Man.
Here's the question: how are you going to fulfill your purpose if you're not healthy? If you're not physically, emotionally, mentally, spiritually, financially healthy, how are you going to accomplish your purpose if you can't get there? Here's is why that's important: It makes it more difficult, for sure, and in some cases, it would be impossible to accomplish your life's purpose if you aren't healthy enough to try. So this book will examine these four things: how to be healthy physically, mentally, emotionally, and this chapter is about what it is to be a spiritually healthy person.

You say, "Well, I go to church." Okay… the old joke is… "Going to McDonald's doesn't make you a hamburger and going to church doesn't make you a Christian."

Being a spiritually healthy, mature person is different than I just go to church or I go to a small group. It has to do with the way the things of God influence your life.

The guidelines in the Bible are not fences; they are guardrails designed to protect us.

THE GUARDRAIL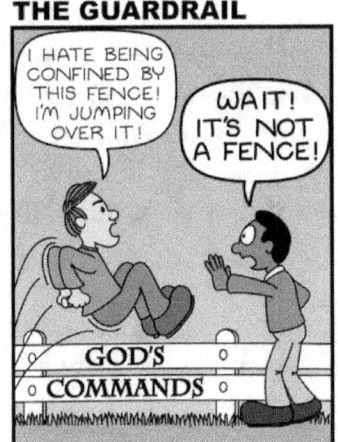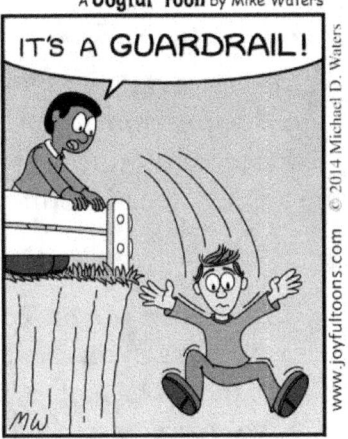

A **Joyful 'toon** by Mike Waters

Whoever keeps commandments keeps their life,
but whoever shows contempt for their ways will die.
– PROVERBS 19:16 NIV

Here's number 1: *A spiritually healthy person understands the Biblical perspective of the spiritual condition of mankind.*

I run into people all the time that say, "I think mankind is basically good." Okay, I guess that could be true. Mankind does do some really good things.

However, that's not necessarily the Biblical perspective of the spiritual condition of mankind. And it's not a bad thing to admit that the Bible could be [and is probably most likely] definitely right.

Romans 3:23 says, "All have sinned…" Not most, not all the people over 20, not all the people over 6, it's says everyone has sinned and we fall short of God's ideal for what He wants for us. That's what it means to fall short of the glory of God. And at some moment, everybody everywhere on the planet has goofed up. *We've done something less than what God intended for us to be and do.* And so God wants us to be holy, He wants us to be righteous. We talked about this in the marriage series. We want to be right. God wants us to be righteous. And there's a complete difference.

1 John 1:8 says, "If we say we don't have any sin, we deceive ourselves." *I hate to tell you this but you are your own worst enemy. We are our own worst enemy.* **We bluff ourselves into believing and doing things, which we know are not true and not right.** But we bluff ourselves into believing that it's correct. It says we deceive ourselves and "the truth is not in us."

In other words, inside of you, imagine, Jesus [represented by the Holy Spirit] lives in one half of you and you [our sinful nature] live in the other half. When we do what Jesus wants, chances are we're going to do what's right because the Spirit of God is in control. When we crowd Jesus out and we do what we want, that's when we sin. And I hate to tell you this, but Jesus and sin cannot live in the same house. He doesn't like it. He's uncomfortable there, in the presence of sin.

You may say, "Well, God is everywhere." Well, from a Biblical point of view, no He's not. *God is not in sin.* **Because God and sin don't go together.** So when there is an act of sin, God is not in that act *because it violates His character.* If we deceive ourselves, and say we haven't sinned, we're kidding ourselves. The truth is not in us. Our side has crowded Jesus out at that moment to do what we want. If we say we haven't sinned you're just fooling yourself.

Keep in mind that "sin" is a single act. I sinned. I told a lie. I stole something. Those are single acts. I sinned. For all have sinned. Everybody everywhere has done at least one thing wrong. I don't think anybody can get up front, any place anywhere and say, "I have never goofed." That goes for Pastor Tom, all the Pastors here, every person walking the planet, everybody has goofed.

However, it's completely different to be sinful and to be defiant in everything. Those of us that have kids, it's one thing for your child to do one thing wrong. It's another thing for your kid to be totally defiant. Right? So an attitude of defiance is completely different than, "I did one thing wrong." So when you talk to your child, have you ever said this, "How many times do I have to tell this?"

It's one thing to be defiant. It's another thing to sin. And it's another thing to make a mistake. I goofed. I didn't mean to. That doesn't mean that what we did was not wrong. But it's a goof. To be defiant is completely different.

And this is how the Bible describes us. *It describes us as being defiant against God.* Our human nature and the Spiritual nature do not get along. It's a fight between two enemies battling each other. There are two lions at war inside of you and whichever of those lions you feed the most is going to win. And if you feed your earthly human carnal side, as the Bible would call it, if you feed that side of you, that side will win. If you feed the spiritual side of you, that side will win. If you think about, dwell on, listen to, read about, holy, spiritual, righteous things, you are more likely to become a holy, spiritual, righteous person. If you continually fill your mind and heart with other things, chances are that's who you're going to become.

Look at your ten best friends. Rate them on a scale of 0 to 10. *You are the average of your friends.* Why? Because they represent total opposite perspectives. Some of them are 3's. Some of them are 4's. They're not all 9's. And if they are, I want to meet your friends. If you're honest, you're the average of your friends because they have a push and a pull on you. And the people that pull you to the spiritual things, that's how you're going to gravitate. Chances are you'll become a spiritually minded person. But the people that are pulling you to the earthly things, chances are you'll become earthly, worldly-minded. It's just human nature.

And so inside of us, we are rebellious against God. *You and I are rebellious against God.* Some of us learn to taper it off early on in life. And some people are more likely to be spiritually minded than other people. This 'God awareness' happens easier when we're young. The statistics say that 85% of the people who become Christians do it before they're 18. Why? *Because their minds are still pliable and open.* Once you go to college or once we get married, we think we know everything. [All you have to do is talk to your spouse and you'll realize you don't know everything.]

But sinful means [doesn't mean that we make a goof] that we are more likely, given the chance of having a choice, *we're more likely to do what we want instead of what God wants.* That's all sinful means. This is not meant to hurt your feelings. "Oh my gosh, the Bible thinks I'm sinful." Listen, you don't go to the doctor and the doctor say, "I think I know your condition but I'm not going to tell you the truth. You have a headache." You want the doctor to tell you the truth. And according to the Bible, we are sinful people. We are prone to do what we want rather than what God wants.

This simply indicates is that you and I love our way. We want to do what we want to do. I saw something the other day, a sign that said, "If you're doing something fun, you're probably living in sin." [BTW, you can have fun and not live in sin.] But if sin wasn't fun, who would do it? If it was painful, and it separated you from God and people, and it really pleasant, .no one would do it! But sin is fun. Just like other things are fun, too. We get to choose our activities of where we're going to go have fun and who we're going to have fun with. We're prone to do what we want instead of what God wants.

John 3:19 tells us why this happened. "The light…" meaning Jesus "…he came into the world but men loved the darkness." We loved our own way. And this is right after John 3:16 – "For God so loved the world…." Jesus came into the world but men loved the darkness. Men loved to do what they want to do. Humans, mankind is against God. It's actually to the point where in James 4 it called us an enemy of God. Now militarily, that's a bad place to be. You don't want to be the enemy of the biggest, meanest bully in your school. You don't want to be the one that everybody at your work is looking out for and they just can't wait to pin you against the wall. You're afraid of those people. And we have mankind who defiantly stands before God and says, "I will be God of my life. I will be king of my throne." And yet it is God who looks at us and says, "Don't do that. Because in the end I win. You lose." How'd we get there?

Way back in the Old Testament, there was a prophet named Jeremiah who preached for many, many years. The Bible says 40 years. It means a 'generation.' He preached for along time. No one ever listened to him. No one ever turned to God because of his ministry. He's known as 'the weeping prophet.' And what he says here is true: "Above all else, the heart is deceitful." Your heart will lie to you. Your heart will lie to other people. And in fact, when you do lie to other people, it comes from your heart. It's a desire to protect yourself, it's a desire to avoid responsibility. But it's your heart that's deceitful. Now this is not your heart, like the beating thing in your chest. Your heart is similar to that little thing that kids play with, the rock-a-stack. It's got the yellow spindle and the multi-color donuts? The yellow spindle is your heart. *Your heart is your emotions, the seat of how you feel, the seat of how you're committed to things, the seat of your convictions. Your heart overflows every other area of your life and your natural human nature is bent against God. And so everything flows from you being a spiritual person. And if your spindle, if your heart, is not seeking God, every decision you make is subject to you doing what you want instead of what He wants.*

The core that makes you a spiritual person is *your will*. We have to choose to want to follow God. We have to choose to follow God. We have to choose to choose to deny ourselves. We have to choose to follow God. Your spindle is your will, it's your heart. And at the very essence of who we are, we are sinful people. Carnal people. And a healthy spiritual people understands this. And it's okay to say "I'm a sinful person." *It's not okay to stay there.* But it's okay to admit it. So many things keep us from God. All of them are choices that we make. Our ego, our pride, the way we think, the way we act... they keep us from God.

A Spiritually Healthy Person Understands That Our Sin Separates Us From God And Each Other

First Timothy 2:3-6
[3] For this *is* good and acceptable in the sight of God our Savior, [4] who desires all men to be saved and to come to the knowledge of the truth.[5] For *there is* one God and one Mediator between God and men, *the* Man Christ Jesus, [6] who gave Himself a ransom for all, to be testified in due time,

Number Two: A spiritually healthy person understands that our sin, our mistakes, separate us from God and each other. The sin that separates you from God also, most likely, has separated you and I from each other. It's hard for me to do something against God that somehow doesn't affect the relationships that I have with people. And that's why here at Friends we say our goal is 'to connect people to people, and people to God' because chances are *if you're in a right relationship with God, you're going to be in right relationship with each other.*

But our sin, the choices we make, causes us to be separated from each other. "This is a good thing, acceptable in the sight of God our Savior. God desires that all men would be saved, come to the knowledge of the truth." That's what God's will is. Part of His Will is that every person, you included, would be saved, saved from living for yourself and instead living for Him. So there's only one mediator. One God, one mediator between God and man, and that is the man Christ Jesus. How do you make amends with God? The answer is Jesus: He is the One who said, "I am the Way." He said that there is One way to get to God.

"Well, that's not what the people who knocked on my door said." I have a lot of people knock on my door. Most of them are selling something. Lawn care. Alarm system. Have you heard this one yet? "I was just in the neighborhood, and about 35 of your friends…" Really? Can you give me their names? "Oh I'm not allowed to do that."

These people that knocked on my door said that's not how you get to heaven. *They could be wrong.* I'm just saying. They could be wrong. *Because the Bible says, and makes it clear, that the only way you get to God is through Jesus Christ.* Who is He?

"He gave Himself as a ransom for all to be testified…" [that means acknowledged, realized, recognized, in due time, sooner or later, you can pay me now or you can pay me later, but you're going to pay Him…] "Every knee will bow" is what the Bible says.

"He gave Himself as a ransom." Now I really like Eugene Brown, our youth pastor, [especially without the beard…it's looking good!] If somebody kidnaps Pastor Eugene, they will want a ransom. They're going to want money. And we're all going to pitch in. It's $14 and some change. Becca's [his wife] has $6. So we've got to come up with $8. Somebody's got to pay to get Eugene back. [Let's take an offering….]

Your sin, my sin, has made us property of Satan. *Somebody had to pay to get you back. And so Jesus paid for you to get you back.* Now keep in mind, you were created, the Bible says, [all creating was done by Jesus,] you were created by God, breathed His Spirit into you, you belong to God in the first place, *but somehow your sin has separated you from and now Satan is the one directing your path.* **But Jesus paid to get you back on His team. Why? Because He wants you, of all people, to spend eternity with Him.**

He gave Himself as a ransom for all… it doesn't say "for some." It's for all. Even the people who hate Him. Even the people that teach against Him. Even the people who don't believe in Him, He gave Himself as a ransom… gave Himself a ransom for everyone that in due time He will be recognized as the only way to get to God.

The Bible says that every famous person will bow to Jesus. It says that every great athlete will bow to Jesus. Every politician, musician, actor, actress, author, TV personality and philanthropist, will bow to Jesus. Everybody everywhere is going to bow. It doesn't matter if you love Him or not, the Bible says "at the time of judgment", we will bow and acknowledge to Jesus, '**You** are the man. I am not. You are the king. I am not.'

My question is, if you're going to bow later, why not do it now and make it easier on yourself? He gave Himself as a ransom.

Probably the most famous verse in the Bible. "God so loved the world that He gave His only Son that whoever would believe in Him…" [By-lieven: By the their lives demonstrate] that they believe in Him… "will not perish."

But here's the next verse. "He did not send Jesus into the world to condemn the world." Some people think God is mean and He only sent Jesus here to make us look bad and make us feel bad. But that's not what the verse says. "God sent Him [Jesus] into the world, so that through Him, [the culture] the world, could be saved." This was a suicide rescue mission to save me, to buy me back, because He loves me. That's why He did this. Not because it looked good. He did it to get you back.

This is what it says in Corinthians. "For the love of Christ compels us, because if one died for all, then everybody died. And if He died for all, those who live should no longer live for themselves but should live for Him who died for them and rose again. So therefore, from now on, we regard no one according to the flesh, even though we have known Christ according to the flesh, we now know Him like this [no longer just a human being, He's a spiritual being]."

What is it saying? He died for everybody *so that the life that I live now in the flesh* [Galatians 2:20] *I now live by faith in the Son of God who loved me and gave Himself for me.* So the life that I live, I realize because I'm a good steward, [remember Stewart and the boat?] this life that I have is not mine. The life belongs to Him. The life that I have I live for Him. The life I live, I say no to me and yes to Him more because I want to be righteous not right. It all goes together. And when my heart, my will, is serving me, Jesus gets crowded out. And when He gets crowded out, self becomes in charge, and self sins, and my sin separates me from God, and my sin separates me from God and from each other.

"So therefore, if most anyone is in Christ…" [Most anyone?] That's not what it says. "Anyone is in Christ, they are a new creature, old things have passed away." Everything becomes new. Who they used to be is now dead. What they used to do is gone. In the eyes of God it's gone.

"But the old has passed away and everything is new. Now all things are of God who had reconciled us to Himself through Jesus Christ. *And He has given to us the ministry of reconciliation.*" This is the part that's a key. He's reconciled us to Him. And He's giving you and me the ministry of reconciliation *so that we can be reconciled to each other.* So just like God was in Christ, reconciling the world to Himself, He's not imputing His trespasses on them, He's not holding that against them, He has committed to us the word of reconciliation. Remember the first part of this Scripture? I am compelled to tell you about Christ.

So we have to be reconciled to each other. Remember my purpose? My purpose says I'm going to have a great time influencing people toward the Kingdom of God. If you don't want to go to His Kingdom, okay. I do want to go. And I want you to go. But if along the way it means I upset you. I'm sorry. I really am sorry. But I have to do what I have to do. I'm compelled to tell you that God loves you.

Christ is reconciling the world to Him and us to each other. You and I have been given the ministry of reconciliation. Those people that you work with that you don't like… [you know who I'm talking about…] your job is to be reconciled to them and to reconcile them to God. It's easy with people that you get along with. That's easy. The Bible said, "It's easy to love the people that love you. But love your enemies." So those people that you work with that you don't really like. Those are the people that you're to be reconciled with. "Oh but they don't want to be reconciled with me." Notice, there's a difference. That description is not reconciled, that's restored.

Reconciliation is a bridge, I'm going to build a bridge to you… that's reconciled. Even if this is a person who does not like you, or that you don't like, you can build a bridge to them. You can invite them to come back across the bridge, If they say no, you did your part. If they build a bridge back, *then the relationship has been restored..* Reconciling is one way, one direction. Notice that the Bible doesn't say, "Wait for them to do something before you're reconciled." It says be reconciled even if they don't want you, even if they still don't like you. It doesn't matter. Be reconciled to them. Invite them across the bridge. And if they don't want to come, you did your part. Reconcile them to God, invite them, show them the path. Invite them across the bridge to you. Reconcile them to God, reconcile to each other.

When you and goof, it separates us from each other and God. We're spokesmen for God. In fact, the Bible says we are ambassadors. Ambassadors for Christ. Just like we're pleading through us… we implore you… that means beg, we beg you on Christ's behalf, be reconciled to God. That is our calling. Why? Because He made Him, Christ, who knew no sin. He put our sin upon Him so that we could become righteous… not right… righteous in Him.

A Spiritually Healthy Person Understands The Biblical, True Nature of God

They don't think that just because we think that God is XYZ, that's not necessarily what the Bible teaches. There's a part of God that's very firm. God's like a quarter. One side of it is love, one side He's just. He's fair. One side is just. One side is love.

What this means is that there are rules. God has rules. This doesn't mean that He's mean. *It means He loves us.* You and I have kids. If you've ever had neighborhood kids, your house had its own rules. And you had rules because you loved them. And they weren't allowed to just come over to your house and do whatever they wanted to do. They weren't allowed to run around and do whatever they wanted to do. They weren't allowed to hit people. They weren't allowed to bite people. You have rules. We don't have rules because we're mean; we have rules because we love people and we don't want people to get hurt. Right? God is the same way. God has rules because He loves us. It's not because He's a big mean ogre and He wants to thump us in the head and prove how big and mean He is.

It says here, 1 John, "Love one another because love is of God. Everyone who loves is born of God and knows God. But if you don't know love, you don't know God, because God is love." *A spiritually minded person understands that if God loved me, I'm supposed to love everybody else.* I'm just a tube. I'm a straw. I'm just a piece of bent elbow macaroni that God just flows through. That's all it is. In other words, if this has been given to me, I'm supposed to give it away. I'm not supposed to hold on to it for myself.

You're supposed to find a way to love other people because God has loved you. "In the love God had showed [manifested, brought to reality] with us, God has sent not only His begotten son into the world that we could live through Him but in this love [it's not that we loved God but that He loved us] He sent His son to be the propitiation [that means substitute] for our sins." God has been really, really nice to me. I'm supposed to be really, really nice to other people, those ones that I'm building the bridge of reconciliation with. The ones I don't really like. Because if God so loved us, we should love the people we agree with. Oh wait it doesn't say that. We're supposed to love one another. That means the people of faith. But it also means other people.

Until the power of love overcomes the love of power, there will never be peace on earth. Look at what's going on all over the planet. You have to have love and demonstrate and show love to other people.

This is from Corinthians 13… "Love [God] is patient. God is kind…" This is truly the definition of God. However the spiritually minded person gets beyond even that to understand that it's through Christ mankind is forgiven. That's it. I can't earn it. I can't get it. I can't buy. Even with a coupon. There's no buy one get one free. "Whoever calls on the name of the Lord can be saved." "But there are some people, Pastor Tom, that cannot be saved." That's not what that says. It says "whoever." And that guy or girl that's in your life that's so anti-God right now, they can still be saved. They're not beyond the reach of God.

You and I are created to do great things for God, created in Christ Jesus for good works which God has prepared before hand so we can walk in them. Those things that you do for God, you're worried about, "Well, I don't know if I can handle this, I think this is above me. I don't know if I could ever get there. I'm not sure this is right." *Look, those things you're doing for God, God planned them before you were born. God laid them out in front of you, He's made a way for you to get there, before you ever breathed your first breath. When He sat around and put one of these and one of those together to make you, your life was laid out in front of you to do good things. To accomplish kingdom thoughts, kingdom principles, kingdom processes. Why? Because He loves You!*

Lastly, a spiritually mature person understands what forgiveness is, how to get it, and how to give it. Thirty years I've been doing this and I meet Christian people walking around all over the place who have a hardness and bitterness and they hate somebody. I'm here to tell you that is a spiritually immature position for me and you. *If I have been given grace and shown mercy, I am supposed to show grace and show mercy.*

"If you confess with your mouth that Jesus is Christ, you believe in your heart that He was raised from the dead, you'll be saved." That's what the Bible says in Romans 10. But it also says, "With the heart you believe and are made righteous, by your mouth you confess and are saved." When you stand in front of the preacher, the guy asks you, "Will you take her to be your wedded wife and, so on. " If you say, "eh….whatever." You're in trouble, in a lot of ways. You have to confess with your mouth. The pastor even says, "You stand here before these witness to confess your faith in your love, one for the other." And you have to say, "I will." And if you don't, it doesn't count. Doesn't count. So your mouth is important. You've got to confess it with your mouth.

"If we say we have no sin, we deceive ourselves, the truth's not in us." We already went there… "But if we confess our sins, He is faithful [He can be depended upon] to forgive our sins and cleanse us from all unrighteousness." What's the point? If you tell God you're sorry, He's really going to forgive you.

"You know, Pastor Tom, I've been praying about this for 13 years. You know one time when I was in the 8th grade, I stuffed a kid in a locker and I really feel bad about it." Listen, God forgot about that in the 9th grade, the first time, when you prayed about it. You've been walking around feeling bad about it all these years, not God. God's like, "What? No, that's done." [BTW, the kid is still in the locker, you should probably go let him out.] If we say we haven't sinned, we call God a liar. Again, bad idea. We say He's a liar, the Word's not in us.

Now here's the pastor part… you remember, "I'm trading my sorrows…" and we're talking about 'sorrow' like 'my sadness'. *Sorrow can be a good thing when you start to think about and it causes you to feel something.*

"If I caused you sorrow by my letter, I don't regret it." This is from the Apostle Paul. [Mr. Total Choleric. Mr. Accomplish the goal, run over people, don't really care. That's him.]

"Though I did regret it for awhile, I see that my letter hurt you, but only for a little while. I'm happy because your sorrow led you to repentance." That's the pastor's job. That's my purpose. My purpose is to lead you to repentance. To each other and to God. That's my job. It'd be great if I could just get up here and give you the big rah-rah speech every week. Set new goals! Love each other! Woohoo! Whatever. But the trouble is, that doesn't work.

The job of the pastor is to bring you sorrow so that you repent. That's what it says. "Because godly sorrow [trading my sorrow] brings repentance that leads to salvation. And it leaves no regret, but worldly sorrow brings death." It's okay to say, I haven't measure up to what God wants. It's okay. And it's okay to say, I've got things I've got to iron out with God. "Because godly sorrow has produced this in you.

A mature, spiritually minded person lives the truth of Scripture. That's what makes a spiritually minded person. These things you read, these things you hear, they don't just go in one ear and out the other. *They change the way you live because they're designed to build up your righteousness so that you can become righteous before God, defeat your humanness so that you can be a spiritually minded person.* That's how you become spiritually healthy: put the Bible into action.

Inside each of us, there's a war. And it's my will against God's Will. It's me against Him. Pay Him now, pay Him later, but you're going to pay Him. And I'm asking you today, commit yourself to being a spiritually minded person.

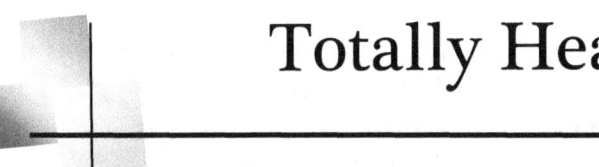

Totally Healthy

On Purpose

What Does It Mean To Be Mentally Healthy?
(This Section was led by Pastor Vinny Korb)

Pastor Tom has shared his purpose statement with you and I think it's important that I share mine as well. My purpose is this: "To love God and to love people by being aware of where God is working and then being faithful to join Him in His work."

I've created a chart that explains this. I call it the "Tuftstonian Quadrilateral of Total Health". It was named after the great theologian T.F. Tufts back in the 21st century. [I don't know where I found this photo. I was very fortunate to come across it this week. But as you can see it's very old. The ends are worn and everything.]

A very good theologian came up with it back in February of this year. But this is the chart. The chart means that each of these components, emotional, physical, mental, spiritual health… they all effect each other. If you're not completely healthy spiritually, it's going to infect your mental health, your emotional health, your physical health. They all interact with each other.

So spiritual/mental, mental/spiritual, so on and so forth. If one is out of order, they're all going to be affected in some way. In order to be completely healthy, we have to achieve health in each of these areas. ...Not that we can achieve complete and total, 100% health. We're imperfect people. But we can always do more to strive towards getting there.

Let's look at "mental health." Let's base this discussion on Philippians 4:4-9 which says this: "Rejoice in the Lord always. Again I will say, Rejoice! Let your reasonableness be known to everyone, the Lord is at hand. Do not be anxious about anything but in everything, by prayer and supplication with thanksgiving, let your requests be made known to God. And the peace of God which, surpasses all understanding, will guard your hearts and minds in Christ Jesus. Finally brothers, whatever is true, whatever is honorable, whatever is just, whatever is pure, whatever is lovely, whatever is commendable, if there is any excellence, if there's anything worthy of praise, think about these things which you have learned and received and heard and seen in me. Practice these things and the God of peace will be with you."

What I want you to know is this: everyone here today can learn the biblical perspective of mental health by understanding these four principles that I'm going to introduce.

The first thing that Paul says here in verse 4:4, "Rejoice in the Lord always. Again I will say, Rejoice!" The first thing he tells us is to rejoice. This past week, my grandmother, I called her Oma, [that's german for grandma,] went to go be with Jesus. This is a good thing. She died but she went to heaven and now she's with Jesus. She was in the hospital from the week before.

Her condition progressed and worsened on Monday. Nicole and I got called to come down to Tampa and say goodbye. When we got down there, we were informed that we were waiting for the doctors to come and remove her from all support.

This was one of the most difficult and one of the most beautiful moments of my life because my family and myself all surrounded her, we stood around her in a semi-circle, and we had the privilege of watching her pass away, which was tough. But at the same time, though we were grieving, though we were in pain, though we were suffering, there was joy. The joy gets its source in Jesus Christ and we knew that her fate was sealed in Jesus Christ. We knew that she had believed on His name and confessed it with her mouth, that she would be with Jesus later that day. So there was nothing to worry about for that reason.

It was tough in one respect, but in the same respect, there was a lot of joy. And the family being there together, there was an element of joy. If she hadn't had such a positive impact on our lives, there wouldn't have been all that sadness.

When you're a Christian, there is always joy. And that's because of where we get that joy from, it source is Jesus Christ.

Joy does not equal happiness. It's a deep contentment in all circumstances. William Barkley says it like this, [and I love this...] "Christian joy is independent form anything on earth because it has its source in the continual presence of Jesus Christ."

So regardless of our worldly circumstances, we have joy, because it comes from Jesus. Keep in mind that Paul wrote these words from prison. We don't know exactly where he was. He could have been in Ephesus; he could have been in Rome. We do know that he was awaiting trial and that he faced execution.

And one of the reasons I think God purposed this, there are many reasons, but one of the reasons that God purposed this, Paul being in prison while writing this, *was to give him authority over what he was saying.*

If he were to say, "Listen, Philippians, I know you're facing opposition, I know you're facing persecution, possible martyrdom, I know you're facing all these things… but I'm chilling over here on the beach in Crete, but you guys, it'll be okay. Rejoice. Thumbs up."

No, Paul was going through these things himself. And that's what gave him authority to write these things. He's saying, "I know what I'm saying. I know you guys are facing persecution and opposition and all these things, that this faith is going to end up in death. Physical death. But not complete death. Because you're going to be with Christ and that's far better. I know what I'm saying. But rejoice. I'm facing these things as well."

So what are some of the things Paul rejoiced in? Paul rejoiced in his imprisonment. That might sound odd to us. Going to prison doesn't sound very good to man of us. But Paul saw it as an opportunity, as a mission field. As an opportunity to preach and proclaim the name of Jesus Christ to the people that were around him.

And many of the fellow inmates were converted because of the preaching of Paul. Many of the guards were converted because of the preaching of Paul. It's difficult to see the joy in that circumstance from a worldly perspective. But from a godly perspective, it's an opportunity. And we have this same opportunity. Though we're not necessarily in prison, but in the work place, in our every day lives, in our neighborhoods, we have the opportunity to preach and proclaim Christ. And we should [as Christians] that should be our mission. Regardless of where God has planted us, we should be willing to share Christ where we're at. Because that's what God wants from us. Paul is saying here to rejoice in all circumstances.

The next thing that Paul's saying is to be reasonable with everybody. This is Philippians 4:5, "Let your reasonableness be known to everyone, the Lord is at hand." So he says to be reasonable. This is a very difficult word. The word Paul used here is very difficult to translate. The Greeks used it to describe justice and something better than justice. It's very tough to sum up in one word but I think reasonable is good. Just think of it as something that describes justice and something better than justice. It's knowing when to relax justice and introduce mercy.

And a great example of this comes from the Gospel of John from the end of chapter 7 through 8:11. And it's about the woman who was caught in adultery. This is what it says: "They went each to his own. But Jesus went to the Mount of Olives. Early in the morning, he came again to the Temple. All the people came to him and sat down and he taught them.

The scribes and the Pharisees brought a woman who had been caught in adultery and placing her in his midst, they said to him, 'Teacher this woman has been caught in the act of adultery. Now in the Law, Moses commanded us to stone such women. So what do you say?' This they said to test him, that they might have some charge to bring against him. Jesus bent down and wrote with his finger on the ground, and as they continued to ask him, he stood up and said to them, 'Let him who is without sin among you be the first to cast a stone at her.'

And once more, he bent down and wrote on the ground. But when they heard it, they went away one by one, beginning with the older ones. And Jesus was left alone with the woman standing before him. Jesus stood up and said to her, 'Woman, where are they? Has no one condemned you?' She said, 'No Lord.' And Jesus said, 'Neither do I condemn you. And from now on, sin no more.'"

Paul is telling us to be reasonable. Jesus gives us an example of what being reasonable is. Jesus knew in a situation when to relax justice and introduce mercy. There are many laws that were given to us in the Law of Moses. There are many things that, many guidelines, that as Christians we need to live our lives by. But the greatest of all commandments is to love.

So there are situations where… we need to take everything on a case by case or situation by situation basis… and see where we can love. Because love comes first. There are times when we must love first and relax justice, in a manner of speaking.

I had to write a paper for my ethics class a couple of weeks ago, and the teacher gave us two options. One of the options was, your wife comes to you and she's trying on a dress and she asks you the age-old question, "Does this dress make me look heavy?" [There was other language used there. I think "heavy" is a better way to say it.]

What do you do?

We had to look at it in a couple different ways. We had to look at it from a rules based perspective. The rules based meaning, we know that Exodus 28 says we shall not bear false witness. That's the rule. We value those rules over everything else. Therefore, we have to tell you the truth. As we all know, in that situation, being that forthcoming may end in severe physical harm, possibly even worse. So is this a rules based question?

You have to look at it from a consequentialist perspective. The consequentialist looks at things and says, "These are the good consequences, these are the bad consequences, I'm going to respond in every situation with the best outcome possible." And that's the opposite end of the spectrum from the rules based, but at the same time, you're not necessarily telling the truth, [unless you are telling the truth,] but you're looking for the best possible outcome. So in that situation, you're going to do what? You're going to sugar coat things, in a nice manner of speaking. That was one of the perspectives.

The last one is a virtue-based perspective. And I think this is the one that falls most in line with the Christian perspective in that we have to do what? Show love first in the situation. Love supersedes adherence to the rules in a situation like this.

Now at the same time, we do have an obligation to the truth. Paul tells us to tell the truth in love. But, this is clearly a scenario where we're going to relax justice and introduce mercy. [I'm very fortunate. I do not have to worry about that question. Just want to say that... get that out there. I've said too much.]

Classically in my own life, I've been more "rules-based" than anything else. I've been told I see things in black and white. The rules says this, we have to follow this.

Here's an example. At the missions garage sale form last year, it was about the time the church CD came out. So I took some of the CDs over there to sell. And I was told, I was given the orders to sell the CDs for $10. So I was thinking, "I've got to adhere to the rules. I've got to sell these CDs for $10." And a little boy walks up with $5 and he offers it. He says he'd like to buy the CD for $5. I did not handle that situation well, I did not relax justice in that situation. And I said no. The CD is $10. Now I'm very fortunate, very blessed, and I'm grateful to this day that another member of this church stood up and said, "I will accept that $5 and you can have this CD." Here is why: Because that was a great opportunity to exercise mercy and love.

If that little boy and his family didn't know Jesus before, there's a chance that listening to that CD would help to get them there. Maybe God can reach them through that. Maybe it would connect them to our community. Maybe it would connect them to another community of faith.

It was a great opportunity that unfortunately I missed out on but one of you were merciful enough to relax justice in that situation. We have to be reasonable. We have to be reasonable in all circumstances.

A mentally healthy person understands the value of being reasonable because if we are reasonable with people than we do well to love others. And why? Why is Paul telling us to rejoice? Why is he telling us to be reasonable? He's saying, because the Lord is at hand. He's saying the Lord is at hand. What he means by that is… Paul wrote everything with the idea that Jesus was coming back any moment. Immediately. Any second now, God will be back.

We must live with that same perspective. The Lord is at hand. Christ will return. Christ will be victorious. We don't have to worry about that. He's coming back. We can rely on His word. He will be victorious. The Lord is at hand. So we need to rejoice in all circumstances. We need to be reasonable with everyone.

The next thing that Paul says is this. "Do not be anxious about anything. But in everything by prayer and supplication with thanksgiving let your requests be made known to God and the peace which surpasses all understanding will guard your hearts and your minds in Christ Jesus."

Paul is introducing a process here. It's a problem, solution, outcome type scenario. And the problem is this: People are anxious. And what Paul means by "anxious" is being concerned about God fulfilling your own needs. This is specifically what he's talking about. What he's not saying is… this is not freedom to not care. We are supposed to care about and be anxious about the needs of others. Philippians 2:20 speaks to that well. But he's saying do not be anxious about your own needs. And he's echoing the teaching of Jesus Christ from the sermon on the mount.

This is Matthew 6:30-34. "But if God so clothes the grass in the field which today is alive and tomorrow is thrown into the oven, will He not much more clothe you, oh you of little faith. Therefore, do not be anxious, saying what shall we eat, what shall we eat, what shall we wear? For the gentiles seek after these things and your heavenly father knows that you need them all." Here's the key. "But seek first the kingdom of God and His righteousness and all these things will be added to you. Therefore do not be anxious about tomorrow for tomorrow will be anxious for itself. Sufficient for the day is its own trouble."

Paul's saying do not be anxious. We do not need to be anxious. Because God tells us in His Word that if we seek Him and His Kingdom and His righteousness, all of these things will be added to us. He will provide for our needs. We still need to be concerned about the needs of others. But we don't need to worry about our own needs. God will fulfill those. This is Jesus speaking. This is the man. This is God incarnate. He says don't be anxious. If we struggle with worry, we have an issue with trust.

But Paul doesn't just list the problem here. He doesn't just say, "Okay, the problem is anxiety. Now I'm going back to the beach in Crete and chill for awhile." What he says is, here's the solution. And the solution is prayer. Prayer with thanksgiving. Philippians 4:6-7 means that you believe prayer because you trust God.

MR Vincent who's a New Testament scholar from awhile back, he says that "peace is the fruit of believing prayer." And Paul says that we can pray for ourselves. And he says that we can take everything to God in prayer. That there is nothing, no prayer, that's too big or beyond the power of God. And he says that there's no prayer that's too small that it is beneath the fatherly care of God.
I've experienced this in my own life. I've prayed to God about the big things. God, what should I do with my life? Be a pastor. Alright, God, cool, no problem. I didn't realize all that it entailed. Still very grateful for that calling. God, should I marry Nicole? Yes, she's amazing. Guess what? It was a blessing to marry her. It was the second greatest decision ever... the first, giving my life to Christ. God, should we buy this house? Yes, it will be a blessing to you and your family. It's been a blessing.

But I've gone to God with the small things too. Especially when I was a little boy. Sometimes when I'm a grown man, too. God, I'm scared. I need Your peace, the peace that's beyond all understanding. He's there. Nothing is beneath His fatherly care and He provides me with the peace and the love that I need in all circumstances. He does the same for all of us.

God also gives us the privilege of being able to pray for others. And I just want to talk about this briefly. That, a lot of times... I know it happens in my situation and I'm sure it happens with you guys too, especially when people find out that you're a Christian... they will come to you and will share their worries with you and they will share their concerns with you. And they will ask for prayer.

I want to strongly encourage everybody to, in that moment, take that opportunity to pray with that person right then and there. Because it's important. Because God is sitting up there on His throne. He hears the prayers. It makes a difference. And it helps us too. It comforts us. And it gives us that peace that we all need and that we all desire. We need to take advantage of those opportunities because it's a great privilege to pray for others.

Paul says here that prayer needs to include thanksgiving. This implies that prayer needs to be with gratitude. In all circumstances. And it also implies a perfect submission to the Will of God.

If it's 11:30am and I'm sitting in the office and I haven't brought lunch and the thought of a delicious Chipotle burrito enters into my mind, there's a choice there. That's temptation. [I don't know if it's necessarily sinful to desire a Chipotle burrito. It is sinful to desire other things.]

But the example is this... if I reject that thought, I have the decision to, I have the Holy Spirit inside of me, I can resist temptation. I can choose not to sin. If I reject that thought, it's cool. The thought's not sin, the temptation isn't sin. Giving in to the thought, giving into to temptation, that's where sin comes to life.

In this context, if I start thinking about that floury soft tortilla shell, and that delicious chicken, I don't know how they season it but it's so delicious, and they've got the rice and the beans and the cheese and the guacamole or whatever you want on there... the salsa, and it's all... and I think about what it feels like to take a bite and how my taste buds feel in that moment and the warm feeling I get when it reaches my stomach... if I think about all those things, guess what's going to happen? I'm going to speed at 100mph to Chipotle. I'm going to stand in that line that goes all the way out to the parking lot and I'm going to get one of those burritos and I'm going to eat it.

But this is, though again maybe not sinful within the burrito context, but when a thought, a temptation, enters our mind and we give in to that thought or temptation, guess what's going to happen? Action. I start thinking about that burrito, I start flirting with what it's going to be like when I'm eating it and everything... I'm there. The thought becomes action.

Such is the case with sin. A thought enters your mind, a temptation enters your mind. Not sin. You have the choice not to sin. But you can give in to that sin as well. If you start playing with that idea, it's going to become action.

This is what Paul says in Philippians 4:8… "Finally, brothers, whatever is true, whatever is honorable, whatever is just, whatever is pure, whatever is lovely, whatever is commendable, if there is any excellence, if there is anything worthy of praise, think about these things." This is our solution. This is how we're going to get to not giving into temptation. We need to focus on these things. Not just focus, just think on these things. But wrestle with these things. And Paul lists 8 things here.

The first thing he lists is "true". To think on whatever is true. These are the things that will not let us down. For me, an example of that, the best example of that, is God's Word. God's Word is God's Word. It's not going to change. Whatever it says is going to happen, it happens. It's there. We can rely on it. There may be other things that are true in this world. There's definitely many things that will let us down in this world. But if we rely and think on what is true, we're going to do well to access the power of godly thinking.

Second thing is, think on what is honorable. Good way to think of this is that which has the dignity of holiness upon it. God. Is God not the ultimate example of that. Think on God. Think on what is true. You're on your way to doing well to access the power of godly thinking.

He says to think on what is just. That's fulfilling duty to God and to people. This is the greatest commandment. What is our duty to God? To love Him with all of our being. What is our duty to people? It's to love them with all of our being. It's the greatest commandment. That's our duty. Justice is fulfilling that duty to God and people.

Paul said to think on what is pure. That which is morally uncontaminated. We're going to talk more about that in a second.

He says to think on what is lovely. Another word for lovely that you don't hear in our every day language but it translates the word Paul uses well is winsome. It means inspiring love in others. Now we live in a society and culture that wants us to inspire the opposite of love. We live in a culture where if somebody does something wrong to us, what do we do? We want to get back at that person. We want revenge. We resent that person. We allow all these things to effect us and our total being. It keeps us from getting to the peace of God which He wants for us and which we want. But Christians are supposed to inspire feelings of love in each other. And not just Christians, but into the world. And the way that we do that is with our words but more importantly with our actions. By demonstrating that love. Inspiring love in others.

Paul says think on what is commendable. Another tough word to kind of translate here. It means fair speaking. That's what it means but it doesn't give us a very good picture of what Paul is trying to get at here so it's been translated as commendable. It refers to the holy silence that people had among them when they were doing sacrifices. So if we think about it, it's not too far to say that these are the things that are fit for God to hear. Obviously there are very good things for God to hear, praise, and prayer, and all these types of things that are given to Him and give Him glory, but there are also some negative things that we speak every day. I'm guilty of it as well. There are ways that we speak, things that we say, that are not fitting for God to hear. Thinking on what is commendable is thinking on things that are fit for God to hear.

Thinking on what is excellent. That's the high things, the fine qualities, the brave actions. There's a lot of negativity in the world. If we watch the news, there's a lot of negative stories. I think what Paul is saying here is to focus on the good things that happen in the world. Not turn a blind eye to injustice. We want to be concerned with justice in this world as well. But focus on the stories of people loving each other well. This is what he's saying here and not focusing on these stories of negativity.

Think on what is praiseworthy. It's important. Praiseworthy in praise of God. Praiseworthy in praise of us, as long as we don't get a big head in the process. The most important part of this I think is to be able to be uplifted by the praise of others. What does the world teach? Jealousy. You've got that, I want that. Paul is saying that when somebody else is praised for doing well, by God, that we should be uplifted by that praise.

These are the eight things. And godly thinking is focusing on these things. There's power in godly thinking. It enables us to become like Jesus. Now here's the problem. We live in a culture that teaches worldly thinking. I want you to imagine this for a second. It's a hot summer day in Florida. About 100 degrees outside. Humidity's through the roof. You're outside digging holes. And you've been working super hard for about two hours or so. You're thirsty. You're dehydrated. And here comes Pastor Vinny. And I've got a nice tall, ice cold glass of lemonade. But you want this lemonade. You need this lemonade. You're going to get energy from this lemonade. You're body's going to get hydrated. It's what you need. But I've also got a medicine dropper in my other hand. And in that medicine dropper, there's just one little drop of poison. I would never do that to you guys. This is kind of something Satan would do. Like, do you want the lemonade? And then he drops the poison in there. But just imagine for arguments sake. I've got the lemonade, I've got the poison. And I drop that little bit of poison in there.

A Mentally Healthy Person Understands The Biblical Concept of Righteous Thinking

Our society, our culture, our country, I would say over the past 50 years has changed. Evil has always existed. These behaviors have always existed. However, the way that we've looked at evil has shifted. And I would say in probably about 50 years or so, it has shifted. This is what I mean.

One example is that lying is prevalent. There are advertisements on TV where a father is encouraging his son to deceive the mother. And the mother is encouraging the same son to deceive his father. But it's supposed to be cute. It's supposed to make us laugh. It's a picture for how evil has been accepted into our society one little drop at a time. One little drop of poison at a time. But over time, it's filled up that glass and that glass is overflowing now. Another way we see this is is sexual immortality. We've become a morally contaminated society.

Sexual immorality is running rampant. It's not just in the world. It's in the Christian circles as well. Marriage has become an abomination. I'm not just talking about one way, I'm talking about many ways. And the way that we view marriage, there's no or little respect for marriage in our culture now.

Respect for God has lessened. If you think about it, it's not okay to make fun of anyone in this world, or in this country, except for Christians. And it's okay to make fun of God now. I don't think we would have seen that, it wouldn't have been okay 50 years ago. It wouldn't have been acceptable. But there's been a shift.

And this is the thing, I think respect for God is probably the worst thing, but another terrible thing is that love for people has been replaced by indifference. And I think about the parable of the Good Samaritan and I think that the people in our culture, [and I think to a degree we're influenced by that for the most part...] we're more like the guy that walked by the man that was hurt than the guy that stopped, the Samaritan that stopped and helped that person.

We may not think about this being the worst or one of the worst things, but what is God's greatest commandment? To love Him and to love people. If we're not doing that, we're in trouble. In order to access the power of godly thinking, we must commit to think on the things that God values. These eight things that we've talked about today.

So we've talked about the biblical perspective of righteous thinking, we've talk about the power of godly thinking, now we come to our next point... a mentally healthy person understands the connection between the mind and the heart. Christianity's not about what we know; it's about what we do.

"What you have heard and learned and received in me, practice these things and the God of peace will be with you."

It truly matters who we are on the inside. It does matter in the respect that we are in Christ. But what Paul is saying and what that example is saying, all these things you think about doing, that's not what matters. All these things that you know, that's not what matters. It's acting these things out, it's demonstrating love. It's action. That's what God is looking for in each of us.

God doesn't command us to be theologians. He commands us to love people. And here's another problem with our society… we view intellect as being greater than compassion. God views the opposite. God views compassion as being greater than intellect. Paul says these things. He says, "Live out what you have learned from me." What they have learned from Paul is his interpretation of the gospel. This is Paul's preaching. And Paul is preaching based on what he received from the apostolic tradition, the teachings of Christ. "What you have received from me", that's that tradition, that church tradition that Paul has brought through himself and interpreted through his teaching. So what they've learned, what they've received, and what they've heard is part of that as well… But I think this is one of the most important… "What you have seen in me."

Again, Paul is in prison, he's rejoicing, he's using that as a mission field. He's gone all over the known world preaching Jesus Christ. He's done everything he can to preach Jesus Christ. He's not just saying these things and writing letters and sitting here or there… he's a man of action. He's out there doing these things. He's living his life out. And he's saying for the Philippians to do the same, to live this out, and it applies to us as well. We are supposed to live these things out.

Earlier in his letter to the Philippians in verse 2:12-13, Paul says: "Therefore my beloved as you have always obeyed so now not only as in presence in my presence but now much more in my absence, work out your salvation with fear and trembling, for it is God who works in you both to will and to work for His good pleasure." I did a paper on this for school one time and here's the problem… if we're saved by grace through faith, how is it that we're supposed to work out our salvation?

We're not saved by works. The word that's used "to work"…
it means to live it out. It means "to bring to completion".
We're supposed to bring to completion these things that we've
learned. We're not just supposed to get to a certain point and
stay stagnant, call it a day, die, and move on to the next life.
It's not what it's about. It's about moving forward until our
salvation is complete. And as Christians, we should always be
striving towards the standards that God has placed before us.
"Deny yourself, take up your cross, and follow Me."

Paul is urging us to work this out with fear and trembling
because God wants us to live out the Christian way. Not a
suggestion. This is who we're supposed to be. If our mind and
our heart are connected, they need to be intertwined in such a
way that what we know, what we believe is our actions.
They're intertwined like this. They're not separate, they're not
independent from each other. And Paul says to practice these
things and the God of peace will be with you.

There's kind of a little juxtaposition here at the end of verse 7.
Paul says the peace of God will guard your heart and mind.
And here he's saying the God of peace, the peace of God
meaning one aspect of God, but here the God of peace, the
total package, will be with you. Focus on these things. Practice
these things. The God of peace will be with you.

**A Mentally Healthy Person Understands the Connection
Between The Mind and The Heart**

Proverbs 23: 7 For as he thinks in his heart, so *is* he.

Philippians 1:6-8
New King James Version (NKJV)

⁶ being confident of this very thing, that He who has begun a good work in you will complete *it* until the day of Jesus Christ; ⁷ *just as it is right for me to think* this of you all, because I have you *in my heart,* inasmuch as both in my chains and in the defense and confirmation of the gospel, you all are partakers with me of grace. ⁸ For God is my witness, how greatly I long for you all with the affection of Jesus Christ.

A Mentally Healthy Person Is Committed to A Renewed Mind

Romans 12
12 I beseech you therefore, brethren, by the mercies of God, that you present your bodies a living sacrifice, holy, acceptable to God, *which is* your reasonable service. ² And do not be conformed to this world, but be transformed by the *renewing of your mind, that you may prove what is that good and acceptable and perfect will of God.*

So far, we know that a mentally healthy person understands the biblical concept of right thinking, the power of godly thinking, the connection between the mind and the heart… we move towards our final point. A mentally healthy person is committed to a renewed mind. So when we consider the complete segment of Philippians 4:4-9, it's reasonable to say that all these things that are listed by Paul require a renewed mind.
Think about it. Rejoice in all circumstances, be reasonable with everyone, do not be anxious, believe in the power of prayer, trust God, the peace of God will be with you if you do those things, to think on things that are true, honorable, just, pure, lovely, commendable, excellent, praiseworthy, think on those things… not only think on them but act them out. If we do all these things, it requires us to have a renewed mind. Why?

Because we have X amount of years, however old you are, of conditioning, cultural conditioning, and conditioning from other influences as well that teach you the opposite of these things. We need to be committed to having a renewed mind in order to get to this place where God wants us to be.

And that brings us to Romans 12:1-2. "I appeal therefore to you brothers by the mercies of God to present your bodies as a living sacrifice holy and acceptable to God which is your spiritual worship. Do not be conformed to this world but be transformed by the renewal of your mind that by testing you may discern what is the will of God and what is good and acceptable and perfect." Do not be conformed to this world. Be transformed by the renewal of your mind.

All of these things... Philippians 4:4-9... they require us to have a renewed mind. Paul's telling us to live our lives out as living sacrifices, to be living sacrifices to God. To fully submit to Him. When we maintain control over one of these areas, it's called pride. And it's less than God's best for us. We must accept that God's way is best. Paul says we must turn away from the ways of the world, commit to a renewed mind to be mentally healthy from God's perspective.

We are all imperfect humans. We can be healthy but we're imperfect at the same time. Likely, for each of us, as we go throughout life, we're going to have to continue to work on these things. We're not going to get to one area and be like, "That's good. That one's sewed up and I'm going to work on this one now." We have to continually be working at all these things.

The "Great Marriage on Purpose" Series showed us that we have experienced some sort of hurt in our lives. At some point in our lives, someone has hurt us. I've been hurt. You've been hurt. It could have been from a parent, it could have been from a child, it could have been from family member, it could have been from a friend, from a significant other… you fill in the blank. Somebody not even in your family, pastor… whoever. At some point in your life, you have been hurt. When we're hurt, it's human nature to harbor resentment. We either want to get even, or we just push it all the way down and resent that person for a long time. And it can effect us for many, many years.

I am writing from first hand experience. Throughout my life, I've been in a counseling setting 4 times. When I was 13, when I was 19, 27, and last year. It's always different manifestations of the same root problem. But last year I had a big breakthrough. I was experiencing low confidence in my ability to lead people. And I *thought* I understood why that was. I thought it had its roots in being picked on when I was a teenager. But that's not what it was from. It was from something I totally didn't expect. My point is this… I wouldn't have gotten to that breakthrough, I wouldn't have gotten to that point, God wouldn't have brought me to that point if it were not for the help of someone else.

And I want you to know this… we all know it's God's nature to forgive. He wants us to forgive. He wants us to do this, release these things that have hurt us for so long that can continue to impact us that we allow to impact us. He wants us to let it go because He wants us to be at peace. He wants us to experience the peace of God. He wants to be Lord of our lives. And these things keep us from getting there. I want you to know that God doesn't expect you to go through this alone. God provides help.

Depending on the degree, some of us have experienced very traumatic things in our lives, some of us may have experienced things to a lesser degree, but depending on the degree is going to depend on the level of help that we need. It may be that you need to seek somebody out. Maybe you need an accountability partner or mentor. Maybe it's a member of the church family. It may be that you need to get connected with a small group. Maybe you need to speak with a pastor. Maybe you need to speak with your spouse. But we're not supposed to go through this alone. We need to talk to somebody. We need to go through this with somebody. It may be that you need to speak with a professional. There's no shame in that. I was told a long time ago that it takes a very brave person to confront issues in their lives. It takes a weak person to just let it go. It takes a brave and a strong person to confront it and want to strive toward the standards that God places before us.

We all want peace. None of us want to have these feelings of anger and tension and resentment and all these awful things as part of our life. I believe it's God's desire for our lives, it's our desire for ourselves which comes from God, to be at peace. But we allow all these things to get in the way of taking us to where God wants us to be. The God of peace loves you. He loves you deeply. You are His son, you are His daughter, He loves us all the same. And He wants you to experience peace.

Totally Healthy

On Purpose

What Does It Means to Be An Emotionally Healthy Person?

There's a song that says, "Little in me is much like you. In most of me I need more of You." That is such a great description of you and me. Every day we do so many things really, really well. Maybe 95%, 98%, 99% of what we do is great, and then, all of sudden, we fall off the wagon and start to serve ourselves and the next thing you know, we're not being who God wants us to be. And it starts with how we think, then it moves to how we feel. Then all of a sudden, when we don't feel right, or we feel threatened, we start to make decisions that serve me, instead of serving God. And the whole point of this book is to help you be healthy, in all areas of life. In this section, let's concentrate on becoming an emotionally healthy person.

Chances are, the decisions that you and I make will not always be pleasing to God. Can we agree on that? The goal is as we walk with Christ is that more of the decisions, more often, reflect the character of Christ. Would we agree on that? So for us to be an emotionally healthy person isn't dependent upon how long we've known Christ. *It matters that my decision process is becoming more like Christ.* Whether I am a Christian for 40 years or 60 years is irrelevant. *What is relevant is that I'm maturing in my faith and I'm becoming more like Jesus in each and every area of my life.*

Colossians 3

2:1 Since, then, you have been raised with Christ, set your hearts on things above, where Christ is, seated at the right hand of God. **2** *Set your minds on things above, not on earthly things.* **3** For you died, and your life is now hidden with Christ in God. **4** When Christ, who is your life, appears, then you also will appear with him in glory.

A person who is healthy emotionally, they understand how emotions function. Being emotional is not all bad. In fact, everybody here is emotional. Everything we do stems from how we feel. This is from Colossians 3. It's an important Scripture. If you ever want to know about the character and nature of God, the book of Colossians is where you want to go. It tells you all about God's sovereignty.

Colossians 3:1 "Since then, you've been "raised with Christ…"" [Since you're a Christian, is what that says…] "Set your heart on things above." [Remember, we said your heart is like the spindle of the little rock-a-stack. *It's the core of who you are.* From your heart, your will, every decision is made from there. So, "set your heart [set your will] on the things above." Why? "It's where Christ is seated, at the right hand of God. Set your mind on things above, too. Not on earthly things." Earthly things are not evil. But they're not to be our pursuit. They're not to be what we've decided is most important in our minds.

What does is say in verse 3? It says, "You died." I did? *Obviously, I am very alive. However, my will died.* Galatians 2:20: "I am crucified with Christ, nevertheless, I live! And this life I now live in the flesh, I live by faith in the Son of God who loved me and gave himself for me." So we died. Our *will* dies when we become Christians. This is because our will is now hidden inside the Son of God.

Dictionary.com defines emotions like this: "It's a state of consciousness, things like joy, hate, sorrow, fear… these are distinguished from *cognitive and volitional states* of consciousness." In other words, emotions are not something I do on purpose. Cognitive means I've thought about it. I've decided this. An emotion is I love this, I hate this. It just happens. It's not necessarily something that's willful. It is a feeling of joy, sorrow, fear, hate, love, we have lots of emotions.

Dictionary.com continues: "It is a strong agitation of the feelings actuated by experience. Usually accompanied by certain physiological changes, an increased heartbeat or respiration, often overt manifestation like crying or shaking." Like when you were 11 or 12, and you got sweaty palms.

So something happens, I get nervous. Have you ever had that happen? You go to the dentist, you go to the doctor, and all of a sudden, you start getting nervous, you get cold. You get cold because the blood doesn't flow as well. Your hands gets cold and all of sudden you're like, "I'm freezing," and you look and it's 78 degrees in the room and you're cold. You get nervous. Your hands start to shake. You look at someone who's afraid and we wonder, "Why are their hands shaking?" Well, because they've got a fear, something is happening, and now it's causing them to react and act in a certain way.

If you don't know what I'm talking about, imagine your thoughts just before you get on a rollercoaster. Some of us are like, "Woohoo!! Rollercoaster!" Other people are like, "I'm not getting on there." You have to drag those people on there. Some of us love it. Can't wait. Because we're not afraid. Other people are not so sure.

Dictionary.com continues: "An emotion is something powerful, like the emotion of a great symphony." We all have something like a symphony that would cause us to feel this euphoria. These are emotions.

Emotions are a wide range of feelings. However, they start with a thought. You thought about something, and thought caused you to feel something.

And I use the situation here of Saul, [King Saul] and David. King Saul believed that David's mission was to kill him. That's what Saul was afraid of, that David was going to kill him and take over the throne. Saul, would probably be considered... crazy...nowadays. But Saul was convinced. And Saul thought about this long enough, he convinced himself he was right and, therefore, David became his enemy. Saul tried to kill David. And if you remember the story, Saul was out to get David and there was a guy in the middle who was Saul's son named Jonathan. Jonathan would warn David. "Dude, my dad is crazy. You need to go hide. This guy is going to kill you." And two different times, while Saul slept, one time while he was asleep, David snuck up on him, in the middle of the guards, and put his spear in the ground next to his head, which is, "I could have killed you." And the next time, Saul was in a cave, sitting down doing his business, and David snuck in, took a knife, and cut off part of his robe and said, "Could have killed you again." But it was Saul who was nuts. But he convinced himself that he was *right.*

You say, "Pastor Tom, I don't do any of that." Really? How many of you are petrified of spiders? Doesn't matter how big they are, doesn't matter what color they are, doesn't matter where they are, you're petrified of spiders, right? That's why God gave you shoes. And magazines. Swat them bad boys. There's one good kind of spider. And that's a dead one.

Snakes. Some people are like, "Oooh, no way. I don't like snakes. They're slimy." No they're not slimy. "Yeah, they are! They're slimy!" How do you know? "Because I believe it!"

It's a thought, and you take it, and all of a sudden, you believe it's true. And it may or may not be true. How do these thoughts, become feelings? It's because they linger too long. We think about something and we think about, and we re-think about it, and we think about it, and pretty soon, it's so real, we're paralyzed.

I want you to understand, Jesus said to the people, "Don't be anxious about what you're going to eat tomorrow. Don't worry about the lilies of the valley. We feed them, we're going to feed you too." [paraphrase] He's not saying don't be concerned. What he's saying is, *don't be so worried that you're paralyzed, that you don't do something about it.* "Love your neighbor as you love yourself." Remember that verse? So the next time I'm hungry, I'm going to feed me, because I do love myself, right? Whether it's today, tomorrow, Wednesday, I'm going to feed me. Don't worry about it. You know you'll take care of yourself. Don't be so paralyzed, nothing happens.

James 4: 7 says, "Submit yourselves, then, to God. Resist the devil, he will flee from you." Great Scripture from James. But look what it says next. "When you come near to God, He will come near to you. Wash your hands, you sinners, purify your hearts, you double-minded."

What he's saying is, get rid of the things in your life that are causing you to sin and causing you to doubt and causing you to stay away from God. Get rid of those things. And when you go to God, He will come to you. "I've prayed to God and He won't forgive me." That's not what that says. This says that when you go to God, He comes to you. Many other Scriptures... "you will find Me when you seek for Me with all your heart." But you have to want this. You've got to want to be moved toward and be drawn to God, for Him to be drawn to you.

A long time ago, Sherry and I were in bed trying to fall asleep, laying in bed, and all of a sudden there's this big BAM in my house. I thinking, I'm scared. I know I am scared. I am SO scared I am paralyzed. I know there's somebody in my house. I had an alarm clock right above my head on the bed frame, and it put a shadow right on my door.

And I'm thinking, "I'm not getting up. The bad guy will know I'm awake." Sherry said, "Did you hear that?"
"Yes."
"What are you going to do?"
So I said, "Get up!"
"No!"

And I remember laying there, looking at the ceiling, petrified that I couldn't go back to sleep because I was so scared.

Then this verse came to my mind. And I thought, "You know what, resist the devil and he will flee from you." So I start thinking about God, I start thinking of things of peace and things of calm and pretty soon I fell back asleep.

Then there was another BAM and I was like, "Ooooh, no...." There's definitely somebody in my house. I did nothing. I laid there because I was so scared. The next morning, I came out of my bedroom, tiptoeing through the hall, to discover that a plant had fallen over. That's all it was. I was afraid of a plant. That's the truth. *But in my mind it was so much worse.*

This happens when we go to the doctor. We fear it's going to be so much worse than the news we get. Submit your thoughts. Submit yourselves to God, He will come to you.

And it's because our thinking controls how we feel and our emotions control how we behave. And if Christian people are going to change how they behave, it starts with changing how we think. That's how it starts. I've got to change what I'm thinking about because that will change how I feel. And when my feelings are better, my behavior is better.

You say, "Give me an example." This is from Luke 9 starting verse 51. "As the time approached for Jesus to be taken up to heaven, Jesus resolutely set out for Jerusalem." [Resolutely is a great word. I like that. I'm going to go to Jerusalem no matter what.]

"And he sent messengers ahead of him and they went to a Samaritan village to get things ready for him. But the people there did not welcome Jesus because he was headed for Jersualem."

"When the disciples, James and John [the Sons of Thunder], when they saw this, they asked, 'Lord, do want us to call down fire from heaven and destroy them?'" This isn't, calmly, "Lord, would you like for us to call down fire from heaven and just, you know, destroy them?" These guys are hacked off.

"Who are you to close your town to Jesus? Do you know who He is? This is Rock Star Jesus. And I'm one of his little buddies." That's what this is about. This is not about Jesus. *The statement is really about them.* And these Samaritan people said no, the disciples were hacked off and wanted to kill them. On the spot.

How would we feel becomes a door for how we're most likely to act. And if we're going to change how we act, we've got to change how we think.

"Jesus turned to them and he rebuked them." Which is basically, "Would y'all stop it? What you are feeling is wrong."

"And then, He and the disciples went to another village." Jesus behavior was more like this, "Look, if they don't want us hanging around, we'll just go someplace that wants us. You don't have to get all worked up, you don't have to destroy people. It'd be cool to see, but I don't want to do that today. So you guys are in the wrong. How you feel is wrong. Not wrong, as in incorrect only; how you feel is sinful. You're wanting to destroy people that are innocent people. C'mon! If they don't want us, let's go someplace that does." He rebuked them. And they went to another village.

An Emotionally Healthy Person Understands How Emotions Function

What are emotions?

1. an affective state of consciousness in **which** joy, sorrow,**fear**, hate is experienced, as distinguished from cognitive and volitional states of consciousness.
2. any of the feelings of joy, sorrow, fear, hate, **love**, etc.
3. any strong agitation of the feelings actuated by

experiencing love, hate,
fear, etc., and usually accompanied by certain physiological ch
anges, as increased heartbeat or respiration,
and often overt manifestation, as crying or shaking.
4. an instance of this.
5. something that causes such a reaction: *the powerful emotion of a great symphony.*

An emotionally healthy person understands the value of emotions. Emotions are important. You feel in love at some point in your life… you fell in love with that dog, you fell in love with that cat…. [I don't understand loving cats, but that's between you and God.]

Here's some examples:
        When you're feeling threatened, it's your emotions that cause you to want to protect yourself. Fight or flight as it's known.
        It becomes the inspiration for doing something, painting, writing a song, writing a note, your emotions are the motor that gets that going. It's to get you motivated to do something you wouldn't normally do. I'm going to clean my house today.

It's an emotion that gets you going. And it is the response to someone else loving you or caring for you, where it's an emotion that gets you to say okay.

But here's the thing, emotions are also the things that fires up athletes. Talk to these guys who are going to go play in the super bowl or a boxer before they go in, they're ready to go man. They're so motivated, they're off the chart.

People that are in the military, sitting there and they've got bombs going off all around them and bullets flying around them. Why do they do what they do? Because emotionally, they're so engaged. Why do we bring them off the front lines every now and then? So they can recharge. Because they're emotionally tanked. What happens to you when you work 12 to 15 or 18 days in a row? Emotionally, your tank is empty.

Think about the men and women who are first responders. What gives men and women the courage to run *into* a burning building? Because I know what I'd do. I'd run out. Emotion. *They're convinced that it's the right thing to do.*

And when bullets are flying and bombs are flying, those men and women are convinced, "Our military is better than theirs. This gun will protect me. This armor will protect me. This tank I'm riding in is better than anything they have." They're convinced emotionally; in their head they begin to think it and they believe it and it changes how they act. Because emotionally they've got it figured out. This is a good thing.

Healthy emotions are based on healthy thinking. Period. And if emotionally you and I are a wreck, chances are, our thinking is a wreck. And we want to change things. "Oh I wish I could be this, I wish I could do that." *You've got to think differently in order to feel differently.* You have to base what you do on the truth or you are a target to be defeated over and over and over again. Why is that? You've opened the door. You've opened the door to say, "I'm living less than the truth," so you're susceptible to being deceived and being duped.

Here's a biblical example. This is in Matthew 26. This is where Jesus has had the last supper with the boys and now he's heading to the garden. Matthew 26 verse 33, Peter is the courageous one. Jesus says, "Tonight I'm going to die." And Peter says, "No, I will defend you to death!" You can just see him with his little Star Wars Light Saber. Verse 33, Peter says, "I am the man, I will protect you, don't worry about it." And in verse 35, it says, "All the disciples said the same thing." All of them. Peter wasn't the only one who said I will defend you to death. All of them said it, with the exception of Judas. He's already scooted. So we've got 11 guys that are now willing to die.

In verse 70, a few verses later, Peter is afraid of a little girl. This is Peter, the construction worker-fisherman-Harley driving-tattooed-MMA-big tough guy who drives a pick-up truck. This is Peter. The " I don't care who you are, I'll cut your ear off" Peter, the "I will battle to the death" Peter who's all of a sudden afraid of a little, junior high girl. He denies Christ 3 times. The same Peter who said "I'm the man."

Judas is a wreck emotionally by this point. He's seen Jesus be arrested and he's a mess thinking, "Oh my gosh, what did I do." And he was such a wreck, he went and killed himself.

Here is the problem. *They forgot what they were told. **Their emotions were based on their circumstance, rather than the truth.***

Here's what I mean… in Matthew 26:1, 32 verses before, it says that Jesus finished dinner with the boys, and this is what he said to the disciples:

"As you know, the Passover's in a couple of days, and [me, I'm] the Son of man, [I'm] going to be handed over and I'm going to be crucified." *Crucified means dead right?* So He's telling them, "And I'm going to die." He told them, what was going to happen.

And a few verses later, which is probably a few hours later, they'd forgotten what he said. And they're reacting to how they feel.

And then He says, "After I have risen, I'm going to go ahead of you into Galilee." They forgot that part too! So He's saying I'm going to die, really, but by the way, that's not where the story ends. I'm going to rise from the dead, and then I'm going to go with you and we're going to go to Galilee."

But a few moments later, the truth didn't matter anymore and emotionally they were taken advantage of. You have to behave in a way on things that you know are true. You and I both. And the Bible's pretty clear. Think about things which are true and lovely and good report and honest. The Bible's clear. *Because if you don't act on the truth, you're going to find yourself in trouble.*

Two years ago in July, Sherry was working at the Hilton Hotel company and I got a phone call from Hilton. "Your wife has been taken to the emergency room, she may be having a heart attack." Her blood pressure's way high. She's in an ambulance. I tried to call her and can't get through to her, because they don't let you answer your cell phone when you're on the gurney. [Silly rules].

The hospital is in Apopka. FL. Fifteen minutes from her work, forty-five minutes from my house.

I jump in my car. I drive over there. I actually beat her and the ambulance to the emergency room. I'm there *waiting for her to arrive.* [Good thing we weren't in a hurry.]

On the way there, I can honestly tell you this is how I felt: "She's fine." Why? This could be tragic. Could be a massive heart attack. But they didn't tell me that. Could be high blood pressure. They didn't tell me that. All they said was, "Your wife is on the way to the hospital." *So far, I don't have anything to be worried about.*

Do you understand what I'm saying? She finally arrived. Her blood pressure was incredibly high, to the point where she could have, and probably should have had, a stroke. Turns out it was a goofed up of some medications, caffeine and some other stuff.

But here's my point, why be worried, why be concerned, why be paralyzed, *by what I don't know is true?* You don't know what's true yet.

Go to the doctor, find out, and then be concerned. How many times have you and I gone to the doctor and they tell us that it's nothing. Their treatment: "Just do this and it'll be fine."

Sure we are relieved. But we also think, "Oh! I worried about this for ages and I wish I'd taken care of this when I was 11."

An Emotionally Healthy Person Submits Their Emotions To the Spirit of God
Lastly, an emotionally healthy person has submitted how they feel, their emotions, to God. It means "I don't want to feel this way anymore, I want to feel how you want me to feel."

You have to submit your feelings to God. 1 Corinthians 2:14 says "the person without the Spirit does not accept the things that come from the Spirit of God."

Have you ever talked to one of these people at work? You try to tell them something happened at church they say, "What are you talking about?" This is why. You're talking about something that's of a spiritual nature, of a spiritual issue. They don't get it because they don't have the Spirit of God inside them. They look at it and go uh... no, I don't understand. The reason they don't understand is because you're talking a completely different language.

"Oh I prayed about it." You did what?
"It's in the Bible, I believe it." What?

I was thinking about this this week. A person will come and they'll want to debate the scripture with you. And they'll say that the Bible is not true.

It just dawned on me, I was out walking my dog [I have these deep thoughts when I walk my dog] and I'm walking my dog and I'm thinking, "Why is what you said enough to disprove what I believe? If I believe it by faith, who are you to say by your version of "the facts" it's not true?

This is a silly process. It's ridiculous because you've eliminated faith from the conversation. And if you eliminate faith, you've eliminated the spiritual life. Because much of what I believe is by faith. Doesn't it take 'faith' to 'believe the facts,' too?

Listen, it doesn't matter what the news says, it doesn't matter what the TV says, it doesn't matter what the newspaper says, it doesn't matter what your neighbor says, it doesn't matter who comes and knocks on your door, it doesn't matter what they say. *What matters is what the Bible says and what the Bible says will reign supreme in the end.*

And you and I, because we don't know what it says, we don't know how to feel. Because we don't know how to feel, we don't know how to behave. And we live in a culture with people where when you try to talk to them about spiritual things, they say, I just don't get it.

Well, right there is why. You say, well, what else? The best part of that scripture says, "they consider these things to be foolishness. They cannot understand them because they're discerned only through the Spirit."

Isn't it weird how accurate the bible is in describing our culture.? People don't get it. Why? You're talking another language. You're talking a spiritual language. The person with the spirit, "they make judgments about all kinds of things, but such a person isn't subject to mere human judgments."

So in other words, the way the culture feels isn't necessarily how I'm supposed to feel. Why? Because I'm a spiritual person and I'm going to make a spiritual judgment about these things.

How many times have we gone to somebody and said, "Well, I'm having trouble with my kid" and they reply, "Well, this is what I would do." And our first thought is, "Yeah, tell me more. Tell me what else."

"I'm having trouble with my spouse."
"Well this is what I would do."

But what does the Bible say? What does the Bible say about these things?

I'll tell you one thing it doesn't say. It doesn't say for you to wait for them to do something right before you can do something righteous. *Our job is to be righteous long before the world is right.*

And I told you a couple of weeks ago, the world will not be full of the power of loveuntil people quick loving power. The power of love will have its way when people quit loving to be in power.

Man, the Bible challenges us. What's the point? We can have the mind of Christ! Who has known the mind of the Lord? So we can help and learn and instruct him in that way? We can have Jesus's mind. In other words, when I submit my mind, remember I draw near to Him, He draws near to me, when I give Him my mind, His mind can become my mind. And when my mind becomes like His mind, I'm going to do what He wants and so I'm going to do what's righteous. So He's happy and probably I'm happy too. But when I ignore his mind, I'm going to do what I want. And when I do what I want, chances are, I'm going to really, really mess up.

Emotions that are not submitted to the Lord are under the control of self. You're either carnal or spiritual. Every decision you make, you've either submitted it to God, or you've done what you wanted to do. I have either submitted it to God, or I have done what I want to do. Every thought. Every emotion. And when I take my thoughts captive and I make them obedient to the law of Christ and I've set my mind on things above and I've set my heart on things above because that's where Christ is seated with the Father, I'm more likely to do what's spiritual instead of doing what's carnal.

God is always in control of our emotions. Here's the thing… some of you are reading at this and going, "Nooo… that's not always true." God is always in control of our emotions. True or false?

It depends on who God is. It depends on if it's a big G or a little g. It depends on whether it's me or it's Him. But God is always in control. But who's God? You and I have to understand, there's a war between what's spiritual and what's carnal going on in our heart all the time. Every time. Every decision.

And when a thought pops into my mind, if I look at it and go, I know that it is not of God, and dismiss that thought, I haven't done anything wrong. The Bible doesn't say that a tempting thought is sinful. It says to dwell there and to figure out how I could get away with it, now we've sinned, because my will's involved. But things that come in and go out, that's life.

But as a spiritual person, we have to think, "Wait, that's not godly, I need to get rid of that."

Other things that come into my mind, I need to think about that. I need to pray about that. I need to dwell on that. You draw near to God, He draws near to you. Every thought. Every action. God is in control. A emotionally healthy person does what the spirit says.

In Acts 2, the Holy Spirit shows up. This is from Acts 1:8. "You will receive power, the Holy Spirit when He comes on you. You will be my witnesses." [Not go witnessing by the way. It doesn't say that.]

"You will be my witness in Jerusalem, Samaria, to the ends of the earth." In Acts 2, the Holy Spirit comes, the disciples are in the upper room about 125 of them or so. They're hanging out having a good time. They receive the Holy Spirit.

The Holy Spirit comes and invades their lives, the next thing you know, they're believing, thinking and doing things the way God wants them done. In Acts 2:14 Peter stood up with who? The eleven. [Because they've already elected Matthias to replace Judas.] He stands up with all the disciples, the ones who said we will die with you Jesus. Remember those guys? The ones who pledged to die with Jesus?

Now I want you to imagine this. They're in front of a crowd of 3000 people. Were there exactly 3000? No. The point is that there were a lot of people. And they stood up, eleven guys stand up with Peter and they whistle and say, "Hey! We've got something we want to say."

The same coward. The same guy stands up and says, "I've got something to say. We all want to say it, in fact. You guys need to sit down and listen." Do you think he was afraid? You bet he was! Especially those first couple of lines.

"Um, hey you guys…." Finally he gets their attention and you can bet his heart was about to jump out of his chest. Why? He's thinking "These people could kill me. There's a whole lot of them. There's 3000 of them and only like 12 of us. We're going to die."

But he'd come to that point. "It's okay if I die for this." Because what just happened up there in that room freaked me out. So Peter gets up and he starts to tell them about the gospel.

Here is the kicker: he believed the truth, finally. And he lived by it.

The Spirit comes, this is what you're going to do, you're going to go do this, and he's thinking, me? Yeah you! I'm talking to you! And he gets up and he starts doing it. And all of a sudden, pretty soon, he's thinking, "This is okay, because I have the Holy Spirit.
And the Holy Spirit is the one giving me the strength to do this.

The Holy Spirit is the one who gives you the strength to stick in there with your marriage.

The Holy Spirit is the one who sticks in there with your finances.
The Holy Spirit is the one who sticks in with you when you've got health problems.
The Holy Spirit is the one when you can't find a job.
He is the one who gives you the strength.
It's not you. It's not us. It's no one else.
It's the Holy Spirit in you.
And if you're not a spiritually minded person, you're going to fail. The Spirit is the one who gave him strength. And Peter's thought is, "I know the Spirit is bigger than any of these people. The Spirit can take out any of these people."
[Remember a couple of pages ago? They wanted to call down fire, blow them all up? They could still do that.]

And now that they know the Spirit is real, you can be sure Peter was walking around thinking, "Don't mess with me. I will call down fire right now."

He's thinking the Spirit is bigger than anything.
The Spirit is the biggest dog in this fight. And you know what?
That means that if the Spirit is inside of me, I'm a winner because that same dog is inside of me. And I am the winner in this fight.

Peter wasn't afraid. Was he nervous. For Sure.
Was he a little scared? Definitely.
But he wasn't afraid anymore because he knew he wasn't in the fight alone.

Peter's actions shouted, "I have the biggest dog in this fight and that dog is inside of me. And if you kill me, I'll die right now but I'm not going down without a fight. And this dog is going to beat you. Because this dog is the biggest dog in the fight."

You only have to be afraid of succeeding. That's all. That's the only fear you should have. I'm afraid that I'm actually going to accomplish my life's purpose. [Are you kidding? Think about how silly that sounds. I'm afraid I might actually do that.]

Your purpose *is why God made you.* His mission is to see you accomplish your purpose.

We live these hapless, helpless, hopeless lives, and we walk around saying, "Yeah, I'm a Christian. I'm so glad to be a Christian. At least someday I'm going to go to heaven, doggone it." Depressed and sad.

And in some cases, that's what we think. And the whole time, God's looking down going, *I've already given you the Spirit, I've already given you the biggest dog in the fight and you walk around like you've been beat down and like you're just ashamed.*

We are the children of the King. We are the children of the Almighty God. We are the sons and daughters, the royal priesthood, called by the name of Jesus to make the body of Christ.

He's waiting for a group of people to get excited about listening and obeying the truth. And the truth is, there's not a person on your street that we should be afraid of loving. There's not a person in your town we should be afraid to walk up to and say, "I've got the best news, God loves you just as you are." There's not a person you'll ever meet that God doesn't love. Even the ones you don't like.

But we are stuck living our lives beneath our privilege.

And here's the part you need to know. *You can't change the outside circumstances until you change the inside of your heart.*

You can say whatever you want to say about the culture. You can say whatever you want about politics, you can say whatever you want to say about sports, or entertainment, or MTV, or the news or whatever, *but you can't change anything out there until you change what's in here.* You just can't.

And the weird part is sometimes "that out there" isn't supposed to change. You are. We go through all these hoops, and jump and climb and do whatever it is we're supposed to and try and make things better. And the whole time, God is trying to tell us, "It's you I want to change. It's you."

My worst enemy looks at me every day. When I'm brushing my teeth. That's him. And you know what, it sounds weird, but I hate him. There are days I wake up, and I wish that person would just evaporate. And you know how I feel.

And if you're don't know what I mean, then I would suggest that you're not being honest.

You can't change your heart until you surrender that heart to God. You cannot change that person in the mirror until God owns that heart.

Every bit of it. Not most of it. Not some of it. Every shred of it. Every moment. And you can't change your heart until you admit that you can't change your heart by yourself.

How we think, how we feel, you cannot find emotional healing in your life until you realize and admit, I can't do this for myself. It can only happen through Jesus Christ. Only.

Totally Healthy

On Purpose

What Does It Mean To Be A Physically Healthy Person?

Everyday we have to travel around, trapped inside our own skin, go about our business, accomplish the daily tasks [and then some more] and at the same time, 'take care of ourselves.'

Statistics continue to climb indicating that our lifestyle continues to damage, even destroy, our overall health. High blood pressure, cholesterol, heart disease, diabetes and so many more issues attack us from every angle.

And then, when you add the deadly illnesses like cancer, alzheimers, leukemia, kidney failure and others, it is apparent that aren't doing something right. But what is it? What does God say about a healthy person?

[This section is provided by Deb St. Cyr-Paul, Registered Dietitian and Friends Church family member].

When Pastor Tom Tufts asked me to write something about health for a book, I jumped at the opportunity. As a Registered Dietitian (RD) I thought, "well that will be fun and easy." Hmmm.

Two weeks later as I sat with pen and paper in hand to get all the thoughts that had been swirling in my head down on paper, I discovered that writing about the topic of health is a bit more complicated than I originally anticipated.

First of all, one needs to define what area of health we're talking about. Mental, physical, social, emotional, and spiritual are all different areas in which we can experience good or poor health. As an RD, it would seem obvious that physical health would be my area of focus; however, I thought, "doesn't physical health have an impact on mental health which in turn impacts social health? Additionally, doesn't the same hold true in the opposite and with all other areas of health?" So my first dilemma was that it is impossible to separate out physical health from the other areas of health.

Second dilemma: how do we decide what qualifies as good or poor health? In 1946, the World Health Organization (WHO) defined health as, "a state of *complete* physical, mental, and social well-being and not merely just the absence of disease or infirmity." But what about the person who was born without sight and has made it their life's passion to be physically active, eats in generally accepted as healthy ways, maintains a vibrant social life, and is content and joyful living their life in obedience to the Lord? That person has no physical vision therefore one could not say that they are in a state of *complete* physical well-being but does that mean they would be considered unhealthy? In my opinion, far from it! However, according to the 1946 WHO definition, this person would not qualify as healthy.

Dilemma #2.
So as I push forward, it is with these two things in mind: one cannot completely separate the different areas of health from one another, and the picture of good health can look different from one person to the next.

Let's talk for a moment about why it's important to maintain good physical health.

The reasons are plentiful!
  1   Increased energy/stamina
  2   Increased ability to fight disease and heal from injuries
  3   Increased longevity
  4   Increased ability to cope with stress
  5   Improved self-esteem; positive mental outlook
  6   Decreased risk of developing chronic conditions such as osteoporosis
  7   Decreased risk of developing chronic disease such as heart disease
  8   Positive impact on reproductive health and off-spring
  9   Slow the decline in physical function that occurs with aging; maintain independence
  10   Decreased risk of cognitive impairments such as dementia
  11   Because the Bible tells us to

Exploring that last reason a bit further, the Bible passage that comes to mind is

Romans 12: 1 which states: "I appeal to you therefore, brothers, by the mercies of God, to present your bodies as a living sacrifice, holy and acceptable to God, which is your spiritual worship."

If our bodies are to be a "living sacrifice" to God, we need to be purposeful in taking care of ourselves. Note that the Bible did not say our bodies have to be perfect, but rather that we present our bodies as "acceptable" to Him. In order for our bodily sacrifice to be "acceptable" to Him, we must pay attention to the way we treat our bodies and keep ourselves healthy to the very best of our ability.

Again I stress that perfection is <u>not</u> what God requires, but He does want our best efforts working within whatever circumstance we are in. In 1 Corinthians 10:31, we are told, "So, whether you eat or drink, or whatever you do, do all to the glory of God."

Does it bring glory to God when I starve myself to conform to the images the world labels as beautiful? Does it bring glory to God when I eat or drink with complete disregard to the fact that I am gaining weight far beyond what my body frame is comfortable holding?   God has called us to be His hands and feet here on Earth. If we are not in good physical health because of our poor nutrition and activity choices, could this actually prevent us from doing His work?

As you read through the list of reasons to maintain good physical health, think about the impact that some of these things could have on your life. What could you do in your life if you had increased energy and stamina? Would you finally be able to keep up with your very active kids or grandkids?

Could you start and complete that huge project that you always wanted to do but never felt energized enough to tackle? Would your improved self-esteem allow you to go out and meet new people, perhaps work toward finding the life-companion you've always wanted? Would you finally ask for that job promotion that you know you have earned? Could you stop worrying about being a burden on your children as you age?

The ultimate benefit for each of us may look different, but maintaining good physical health gives each of us the opportunity to live our lives the way we want to live them, and not be constrained by unnecessary physical limitations.

Besides the obvious answers of diet and physical activity, what other factors impact our health?

1   The community / country we live in
2   Financial conditions
3   Knowledge
4   Personal hygiene
5   Social environment / social support
6   Working conditions
7   Biology / genetics
8   Access to and quality of health care
9   Culture
10 Our behavior

As with most things in life, there are factors that you can control, and there are factors that not may be completely within your ability to control.

However, that doesn't have to stop you from achieving good health. For example, you can't change your genetics. Diabetes may run in your family and you can't change that fact, but by maintaining an acceptable body weight and being physically active, you may be able to delay or prevent yourself from developing diabetes.

If there are factors that are not within your control, are there ways to work around them? It's important to identify what stands in your way so that you can work toward minimizing the impact of those factors on your health.

The choices you make and the effort you put into developing a healthy lifestyle will have the largest impact on your health.

There are a multitude of books and resources that have been created to teach people how to eat healthy. The same plethora of information is true for physical activity, therefore I will not go into great depth here about how to eat healthy or how to improve your physical conditioning.

Instead, I challenge you to set some goals to improve your physical health and find the appropriate resources to teach you how to achieve the healthiest you possible so that you can live your life the way you and God desire!
The following is a list of resources that you may find helpful in your quest to achieve or maintain good physical health:

Eatright.org   Academy of Nutrition and Dietetics
CSPI.net   Center for Science in the Public Interest
EatingWell.com
MyPlate.gov
FruitsAndVeggiesMoreMatters.org
CDC.gov/PhysicalActivity

A Physically Healthy Person Understands The Stewardship of our Bodies

A physically healthy person understands stewardship of your body.

Read this Scripture from 1 Corinthians 6: "Flee from sexual immorality. Every other sin a person commits is outside the body; but whoever sins sexually sins against their own body."

[Think about this... every other activity, every other thing that you do, is outside your body. But when we sin sexually, it includes our body. And that's what Paul is writing. Keep in mind, he's writing to the people who are in Corinth. Corinth was considered to be one of the vilest places a person could have ever lived. The people there were crazy. And especially when it came to sexual activity, they lived completely without boundaries. Everything was okay. And Paul is saying, don't live that way because you're going to sin against yourself.]

"Don't you know that your body is the temple of the Holy Spirit? The Holy Spirit is in you and you've received it from God. And you are not your own; but you were bought at a price. Therefore, honor God with your body."

God, through the Holy Spirit, inhabits your body, your mind and your physical activity. *What we do with our bodies is a reflection of who God is, what He is, and what He's done in our lives.* So my body belongs to God. The things that I do are God speaking to the people around me. So the very life that you lead speaks of God. The very life that you lead is actually His life.

And I referred to this Scripture previously: It's found in Galatians 2:20, "I am crucified with Christ. But nevertheless, I live." [My body is alive but I belong to God.] "And this life that I now live in the flesh, I live by the faith in the Son of God who loved me and He gave Himself for me." [So what I do is an expression of my worship to God.]

It's awesome for us to sing, "I will give you all my worship." But we can tell, when we leave here, if He has all your worship. The very life that we lead speaks volumes as to whether or not we really are His.

A Physically Healthy Person Is Committed to Being a Good Steward With Their Body

In other words, this body is given to me to take care of because eventually somebody's coming back to get it. Do you remember Stewart? Stewart was asked to drive the ship. God gave Stewart the ship. It was "Stewart's ship." [Got it?]

God gave him the ship, but eventually the Master's coming back to get the ship. And He wants to know, all this stuff, did you take care of it?

God gave you a body. You are the steward of your body. And eventually God's going to come back to get that body. Confused? In the Bible, it says that the second coming when Christ returns, He calls the church out to go meet Him in the air. Do you think you're going to get there by FedEx? He's going to take your body; and the body you inhabit, which is corruptible, will be raised incorruptible, according to the Scriptures. So I get to trade my human, physical body in for a spiritual being that is going to live forever. All of a sudden I'm going to become a soul that lives forever.

But He's coming back to get your body and eventually God is going to ask, "Tom, what did you do with that body I gave you?" And I'm going to say, "Well, first of all, You didn't give me a very good one. We need to talk."

We've all gone through this! We've all had days where we wake up and said, "Why can't I be like that person?"

God's going to ask us, what did you do with your body? Did you take care of it? Taking care of the body is important because eventually He's going to want it back.

If I loaned you something, you should take care of it. And when you give it back… I know this is a weird concept young people… but it should be in better condition than when you borrowed it.

If you borrow my car, or you borrow my shirt, or you borrow anything from me and I get it back, it should be in at least as good a condition if not better condition. So if you borrow my lawn mower and it's full of gas, when you bring it back, it should be full of gas. What a concept. That is earth shattering. It's weird.

God does the same thing. He gives us time, He gives us talents, He gives us treasure, and He gives us a body, a shell, a vehicle to drive around in and He wants us to take care of it. Because eventually, I don't know why, He wants it back. *The reason He wants it back is because it shows whether or not I truly worshipped Him by how I took care of it.*

A Physically Healthy Person Is Committed to Living Within Measures of Self Control and Spirit Control

Colossians 4

[2] Devote yourselves to prayer, being watchful and thankful. [3] And pray for us, too, that God may open a door for our message, so that we may proclaim the mystery of Christ, for which I am in chains. [4] Pray that I may proclaim it clearly, as I should. [5] Be wise in the way you act toward outsiders; make the most of every opportunity. [6] Let your conversation be always full of grace, seasoned with salt, so that you may know how to answer everyone.

Remember I told you in the last chapter: God is in charge of all our decisions. The question is who is God. You or Him?

When it comes to decisions, the Holy Spirit is never going to goof. The Holy Spirit is not going to make a decision in your life that is incorrect. This is because the Holy Spirit is truth. Are we on the same page?

However, when I choose to do what I want, sometimes I'm prone to make a mistake. I am likely to choose what's not best. *The goal of spiritual maturity and health is that some of the things I used to say yes to, I say no to now.* Because I have learned, because I'm mature, hopefully, I have learned self-control.

And those of us that are old, there were things that you struggled with when you were 15, 18, 21, 25 that aren't a concern to you now that you're 50. Now let's be honest and say why: because you're tired! And it takes too much energy to do them. Some of the things that you struggle with teenagers, at 15, 18 years old, they're not even going to be issues in your life when you're 35. But you'll have a whole new set of issues.

A physically healthy person learns to say no to themselves, because the Spirit enables us and because we grow up mentally. We begin to see, that's not good for me. That's just not good for me. A person has to learn to live within self-control.

This is from Colossians 4. "Here's what you do guys," "devote yourselves to prayer," [that's a good idea…] "be watchful," [Pastor Vinny told you in his teaching that Paul believed Jesus could come back any minute… you better be on guard] "be thankful," [the Bible doesn't teach us to be thankful *for* everything; the Bible teaches us to be thankful *in* everything] "and pray for us too" [Paul's in prison, by the way] "that God would open the door for our message so that we may proclaim the mystery of Christ which is why I'm in jail. Pray that I would proclaim it clearly, just like I should. Be wise in the way that you act toward outsiders. Make the most of every opportunity. Let your conversation be always full of grace, seasoned with salt so that you may know how to answer everyone."

In Bible days, salt was used for many things. Salt was money. Because it was very precious, it was considered money. They used it to season food, which we all are familiar with. But they also used to use it to preserve food. Because if you treat something with enough salt, you preserve it, you dry it out. So Paul is saying, "let the way that you talk be beneficial. It's either very, very valuable, it's very, very tasty, or it's preserving the things that are good and natural."

"Let your conversation be full of salt." Interesting word, "conversation". You see, we can tell what you love by how you talk and what you talk about. The same thing goes for me.

When you get me off to the side and we begin to talk and if we meet up somewhere together at a restaurant, it won't be long until I'm talking about Lucas [My grandson]. Why? I kind of like him. He's important in my life. I'll talk about my family, I'll talk about my church, I'll talk about the things that I love to do.

But if you want to sit down with me and talk about things I know nothing about, I'm not even going to be able to carry on a conversation with you. Why? Because I don't know anything about it.

"Let your conversation be seasoned with salt." The word "conversation" in the Greek does not mean speech; it means *behavior*. "Let your behavior be seasoned with salt." So that when others see it... remember it said [be careful with outsiders] be careful how you live, so that when other people see the way we behave, they go, "Hmm... that looks good. That's beneficial. That could help me." The goal is for people outside the faith and see lives seasoned with salt.

Check out Galatians 5, what a great piece of scripture:

"So, here's what I say to you guys, walk by the Spirit and you will not gratify the desires of the flesh."

The left side represents the "me" part of my life. The right side represents what 'God' wants from me. So the left side, these are my decisions versus the right side, those are God's inspired decisions.

The Greek word here for "walk" is actually *"parapeteo."* I actually learned this and it's one of the only Greek words that I remember. And it's because I remember it as "a pair of potatoes."

Parapeteo. In the Greek language, there are several different verb forms. There's one that's a dot. [Something that's never happened before, only happened once, and will never happen again.]

There's also the verb form that it's always been. Always will be. An arrow on both ends.

Then there's the Greek form that it's never happened, there's a dot, and then it goes forever.

And then there's the Greek form which is, it's never happened before, it happens for a little while, and then it stops.

The fifth verb form is something that never happened before, starts once, and goes on forever. And what Paul is really saying to these people is, "Listen, if you keep walking like you are already walking…" In other words, I used to read this and go, if you live by the Spirit, you won't gratify the lusts of the flesh. I used think, aaaarrrghh!

But what Paul is saying is encouraging! "You're getting it right! You've got it down! Just keep walking like you're already walking and you won't gratify the lusts of the flesh." That's what he's saying. And there are so many Christian people that walk around thinking, "How do I get this?" You're already doing it right! Just keep doing it. Keep doing what you're doing. Hang in there.

You will not gratify the lusts of Tom [insert your name here] if you do the things the Spirit wants you to do. Keep walking like you're already walking. The flesh, Tom, desires to do what is contrary to the Spirit. But the Spirit is contrary to Tom. [For sure.] They're in conflict with each other.

Look what it says. "So that you are not to do what you want." Why? *Because what I want is contrary to the Spirit. So don't do what you want.* If the Spirit is in charge, *I can't do what I want.*

I'm angry! I understand you're angry. I want to punch him in the face! Don't do that. Why? That's what you want. That might not be what the Spirit wants. You're not free to do what you want. Man, we've all had times like that, where we're angry, we want to run somebody of the road. You want to call them names, turn somebody in.

Listen, when we do what we want, we're doing not what the Spirit wants. And when the Spirit is prompting you to do something, it's almost always contrary to what you want to do. Because you might look at something and think, "There's no way. I could never do that." Yes you can! The Spirit can enable you to do it.

But the Spirit is going to ask you to do things you can't do by yourself. "If you are being led by the Spirit, you're not under the law." What does that mean? *The Spirit's not ever going to do anything that's contrary to the law.* That's what that means. If you're doing what the Spirit wants, you're probably doing what's right. The Spirit's not going to get you to do something that's wrong, because the Spirit is truth. And what the Spirit leads you to do, certainly there's no rule against that. That's what that's saying. Follow the Spirit. You're not going to have to obey the law, you don't have to worry about it, because you're following the Spirit.

"The acts of the flesh are obvious." Smoking, drinking, cussing, dancing, you know, the big 'sins.' And the reputations continue following people who do these things.

When I was a kid, the list was pretty simple. Outward sin was sin. Period. Inward sin, nobody talked about. That's what this list is. The acts of the flesh, the acts of Tom, are obvious. He lost his temper. Lied. Cheated. It's obvious.

"Sexual immortality [remember, that's where the Scripture started… flee sexual immortality…], impurity, debauchery, [which is just craziness] idolatry, hatred, witchcraft, discord, jealousy, fits of rage, selfish ambition, dissensions, envy, orgies, drunkenness, and the like." It's easy to see those things, right? Right? Those things are easy.

"But I warn you, just like I did before, those who live like this will not inherit the Kingdom of God." *This doesn't mean if you've ever done it once.* Remember, a mistake is once. Paul is talking about a *lifestyle*. If you are totally going to ignore the ways of the Spirit and live by way of the flesh, which is "I don't want to follow God" it means you're not headed to heaven. You're headed to where you want to go and what you've decided to do. That's what he's saying.

But I'm trying to tell you, if you live like this, you're probably not following the Spirit.

"The fruit of the Spirit is love, joy, peace, forbearance, kindness, goodness, faithfulness…" [I want you to notice the word is "fruit."It's not fruits. It's fruit. You get it all. You don't get some.]

"I'm just not very patient. I don't have that fruit." Yeah, we know. But the Word says that you get it all. And you get gentleness and self-control. There's no rules against that. That's what he's saying. *If you follow the Spirit, the Spirit's going to produce these things in your life.* "There's no rules against that. Against such there is no law."

Here's the part that's interesting. When you plant a tree, you don't know when you go to Lowe's and they tell you it's an orange tree, you don't know if it's an orange tree. They could be lying. Some joker could have come through there and switched the tags. You don't know. But you'll know eventually. Right?

And all of sudden, you walk into the backyard one day and it's growing these little fruits on there. And you're thinking, "Ah! This is cool!"

And you go out a couple of days later and the fruits are limes. And you're confused because you are thinking, "I planted an orange tree!" Well, apparently you didn't. You planted a tree. You planted a lime tree. Correct?

You can't walk with Christ for a year, 5 years, 10 years, 20 years, and be a person that has no fruit. It's not possible. You've got some fruit of some kind. And either you have all these fruits, and they may be little bitty, teeny tiny ones, but they're on there somewhere. How do we know? *Because if you have the Spirit, you get the results of the Spirit.*

How do I know? These are things I can choose to do myself or the Spirit works in my life. They're a whole lot easier. I can learn to be patient. I can learn to be kind. I can learn to be gentle.

But you know what, when the Spirit inhabits your life, you can do those things even if you're not wired that way. *Because the Spirit will produce these things in your life.*

"Those who belong to Christ Jesus [that's God's side] have crucified the flesh [that's the other side] and it's passions and its desires. So continue to walk in the Spirit and you won't gratify the lusts of the flesh."

If you have not sacrificed your life to Jesus, been crucified with Christ, this says you haven't committed to Christ. Because if you've committed to Christ, He's in charge of it all. He's a very selfish, jealous God. And He doesn't play second fiddle to anyone. Even you. Even me. If you belong to Jesus, you get Him. It's awesome.

"So, since we live by the Spirit, let's keep in step with the Spirit." You may know that I have a dog. My dog doesn't know how to walk on a leash. She's like 40 feet ahead all the time and pulling at it like I'm trying to water ski. She's this big: 7 pounds! But she just can't wait to get to the next bush or whatever it is. It's like she is thinking, "Come on! Come on!"

So I've learned a trick… walk faster. And you know what she does? Walks faster. I've got to keep in step with the dog. Why? Because it's annoying to me that she keeps pulling me around.

Keep in step with the Spirit. Sometimes He's running, sometimes He's crawling, but He's always moving. And He's moving somewhere. And you've got to keep in step with Him. And I promise you, the faster you run, the faster He'll run. So many Christian people say, "I'm so frustrated! Nothing's happening in my life. I'm so upset with God. Nothing's going right!" Listen, life is one step at a time. Keep in step with the Spirit. And when He looks at you and says, "Come on," and you say, "Oh no, I can't. There's no path." He doesn't have to show us the entire journey: The Shepherd promises you there's a lamo for your feet and a light for your path. A lamp and a light. Just take a step. Keep in step with the Spirit.

"Wait a minute, you have no right to judge me." I'm not judging *you*. I'm judging *fruit*. I'm a fruit inspector. That's a pastor's job. That's my responsibility… to be a fruit inspector.

And I can tell you, over the years, almost 30 years, of being in this business, people just come in and bite your head off, and it's obvious that person doesn't have the Spirit. The Spirit in me isn't saying "Abba Father" with the Spirit in you.

You know what? Christian people aren't supposed to act like everybody else. Christian people are supposed to behave differently than everybody else. Now I will tell you, there's text, Matthew 18, somebody's caught in a sin, the brothers go to him to confront the sin, and help restore them to 'fellowship." I will tell you, in several years of ministry, I've put this process into practice several times in my life and I've never, ever seen it work. And I'll tell you why: *It's because the person that gets called out never responds in the Christian way of "please restore me."* **The church doesn't get the chance to be the church and to see them restored and brought back to health emotionally, physically, spiritually, financially.** And because they get their feelings hurt, or they get their emotions involved, they leave. So the church doesn't get to be the church. So when somebody loves you enough to confront you and say. "You're the man," don't run. They loved you enough to tell you the truth. Go back to them and say, "Now help me. Restore me."

It is what the scripture says. We have a right, as Christian people, to judge fruit in the lives of people. Because there's go tot be something. Even little itty bitty tiny fruit. There's got to be something.

A Physically Healthy Person Is Not a Glutton In Their Behavior

But what is a glutton?

Gluttony. I've been in church 50 years. I've never heard a sermon on gluttony. Most of you have probably never heard a sermon on gluttony either. Well, guess what… gluttony is sinful. It's flat out sinful. *The problem is, we don't know what gluttony is.*

I can remember when I was young, I didn't have any problem with my weight. I was skinny. We're all skinny until 30. Right? And then you turn 40 and you can't get rid of it. And those of you who are young and you're all fit and trim right now, let me tell you, after a couple of kids and a couple of jobs, when you turn 30, you'll be pudgy too. And as I got older, I thought, "I'm not taking care of my body very well. I'm fat. God can't be pleased."

The interesting part was this: I remember reading Scriptures about gluttony and thinking, well, *that's everybody else.* I was talking to a couple of friends and joking we aren't overweight, the thing was "the camera angle's bad. I'm not nearly that big!" Oh yeah, you are. Gluttony is sinful.

But the Bible does not have anywhere sin that is based upon a physical characteristic. Nowhere does it say blonde haired people go to heaven and no one else does. What about bald people?

Or all the blue-eyed people get in to heaven but no one else does.

Or all the people over 6 foot make it into heaven. The Bible doesn't say that. And for something to be sin, it's got to be sinful for all persons, for all time, for all of creation.

Why? In all circumstances, *because God is fair.* He doesn't hold me to something He doesn't hold King David to. He doesn't hold me to something that He doesn't hold you to. So being a glutton would be a physical characteristic that based upon a person's size would be sinful. But that's not what sin is.

Sin, by definition, is a willful act against God. Sin is not a mistake. Sin is when I willfully choose to do what I want instead of what God wants. That's what sin is. So when we look at the issue of gluttony, gluttony's not about being overweight. [I could take you to countries right now where every one of us is over weight. Every one of us.] So every one of us is a sinner? I don't think so. Gluttony is not about being over weight. It's not about being under tall. *And if we are to weigh an exact weight, then it is possible so sin by being to thin.*

What if I told you that almost every person reading this is a glutton according to the Bible in some respect? We are all prone to gluttony. Because a glutton is someone who has an area of their life that is out of control. And that they live in excess. And they live by instinct. I want to feel good. I want to think better. I want to do this. I want to do that. A glutton is a person that doesn't know when to say 'stop.' A glutton is not a person of a certain size.

I know people that eat 7000 calories of food a day, don't gain weight, and they're as fit and trim as anybody you'll ever meet in your life. I know other people that eat 1200 calories a day and they can't lose weight to save their life.

See here's the thing…. A guy who's 6'5" and a guy who's 5'8" shouldn't weigh the same. Right? Just because one guy's bigger. A 5'8" guy at 240 is quite heavy: a man 6'5" weighing 240 is looking quite svelte.

So gluttony's not about a weight, it's not about calories, it's not about a certain size or a shirt size. *That can't be what gluttony's about because then it wouldn't apply to everybody.*

So when gluttony, biblically, means a life out of control, now it applies to all of us. And in some way, when you live a life that's out of control, *something has been placed as more important than God.* It could be finances, it could be exercise, it could be television, it could be vacations, it could be hoarding money, whatever it is, you've placed something in the rightful place that belongs to God, and therefore, you become a glutton.

Look at what this text says. "Many of you whom I've often told…" This is Paul saying, "I've told you guys this before. In fact, sometimes I do it even crying, I do it with tears."

"Many of you whom I've told before now walk as enemies of the cross of Christ." You've been close to God but now you're working against God.

"Their end is their destruction. And their god is their belly." This is Greek for "their God is their own life." They are in charge. God is not in charge.

"And they glory in their shame. Their minds are set on earthly things." Remember last chapter, Colossians 3 says "Set your mind on things above. Set your mind on things above where Christ is seated with the Father." Paul is saying, this group of people who used to walk with Christ, what they're now doing now is what they want and serving themselves. That's not God.

Being a glutton is not about calories. The verse doesn't mention how many calories we should take in. *What the verse mentions is the cross of Christ.* It mentions working for, fighting for the cross of Christ. It doesn't say anything about our physical appearance, what size we ought to be, where we ought to shop. It doesn't say anything about that. It says that what we ought to do is fight for the cause of Christ. He's the one we worship.

You have probably sung it before: "I will give you all my worship. We will worship the Lamb of Glory. I love you Lord and I lift my voice." It's what you sang. "Their God is their belly" when in fact our attention should be the cross of Christ. And that's the one that we fight for.

The verse also says basically this: What are the things that are on your mind? What consumes you? If you were to go home, have 10 minutes to yourself, lay down on your couch, going to take a quick nap, where would your mind go? What would you start thinking about? Chances are, that's your God. Those are the things that are important to you. Because in your times of relaxation and your times of just chilling out, that's where your mind goes. Eventually. These are the things we're consumed with because that's what came to mind first. And a person who is a glutton, whose life is out of control, this is a really good way to determine Who's on the throne of your heart.

Webster's dictionary says gluttony is "habitual over eating." Really? Maybe we ought to look at what the Bible says. That's because Webster does not address the heart issue attached to gluttony. He gives a very basic dictionary.com answer, this is gluttony. And many of us were raised with the idea that gluttony means you're overweight.

I hate to tell you this but 33% of the people in America today are by definition obese. Sugar diabetes, other diseases, are rampant. Heart attack. Heart problems. Off the chain. Primarily, it is because of our food, our overall health and the way we take care of ourselves.

If you have a Bible, take time, get the workbook, you can go through it, in Proverbs, it says, in Proverbs 23, it says many things that are gluttonous.

Here's the difficulty. If can control my eating, and that makes God happy with me, who's in charge? Me. If I can just somehow live a certain way, then God will love me. And if I live this way, but you don't, it allows me to point fingers at you and say what's the problem with you?

"If you were just like me, you could make God happy too." And so what it is, it's all about self-righteous feeling that somehow if I can learn to behave a certain way, then I'll look good to God and God will love me. I don't have to be righteous. I can just be right. And the fact is that if I'm thinner than you, but I'm still overweight, at what level do you become righteous? The problem with this mindset is that it states, "I'm in charge and God is not. And if I learn to behave a way, God will love me." But that's contrary to what Scripture says. It says that grace is given to me as a gift. And it's given to so that nobody can brag about it.

Let me show you something. Gluttony can be anything that takes the place of God in our lives. Anything. Good, bad, ugly. It can be anything that takes the place of God in your life. It's gluttonous because the decision making process is out of control. You're no longer deciding for yourself, you're no longer exercising self-control, and certainly not spiritual control. You're exercising you in control.

This is from Proverbs 23. This is where it says watch out for gluttonous behavior. These are all the things it says in that one chapter.

The first couple of verses, you're better off being dead than being under the control of another person.

Verse 3 basically says to crave and desire to the point of being deceived is not a good idea. In other words, you're susceptible to being duped.

Verse 4 it says don't chase riches. Don't think you're wise. It doesn't take long, the stock market crashes and people lose money.

Verse 5 basically tells us to not be preoccupied with temporary fulfillment. All these fun and games and thrills, be careful, cast a glance at these things.

Verse 6 says don't let your basic needs overpower your character. In other words, I've got these certain needs in my life, but don't let those things become more important than your decision making process and who I really am in Christ.

It says in verse 7, don't be a miser, don't be selfish, don't hoard. Because that kind of person is always looking to take advantage of other people. In the verse before, don't be a miser. Be generous. Don't allow your physical needs to cloud your judgment because this person who wants to dupe you… "Eat! Drink! Be merry! Come on! Have a good time!" And what are they going to do? Take advantage of you. Pay attention.

Verse 10 says don't waste wisdom on foolish people. It's a good thing there are no foolish people walking around. Because they will scorn your words. "That guy's stupid. He doesn't know what he's talking about." Don't waste your time there. That's what this Bible says. Don't be greedy. Don't be deceptive. Don't be conniving. Don't move an ancient boundary stone. So this belongs to that guy. I'm going to pretend, and I'm just going to move it that way. Don't cheat. That's what it says. Don't be greedy. Don't push the limits. Don't go too far. Why? Because the guy whose marker you moved, his defender is God. And God will take up the case against you. That's really a bad idea. So don't do it.

Give your passion to learning, correction, and instruction. Find somebody in your life that's better than you, have them tell you what you're doing wrong, so that you can get better. Apply yourself to learning. It's not just learning. It's applying.

Structure, oversight, and guidelines will lead to success but careless, out of control living leads to death. This is a parenting advice. Children need boundaries. Discipline doesn't mean punishment as in beat them with something. They need boundaries and consequences. Why? Because if you let them live however they want, they're going to probably live how they want and it won't be healthy.

"My son, if you're heart, your will, is wise, then my heart will be glad. My inmost being will rejoice when your lips speak what is right." Now remember, speech is an indication of what's going on in your heart. So my heart is glad if your heart is righteous because you'll talk about righteous things. You've got nothing to hide. That's one of the best things in life is to lay your head on your pillow at night and know nobody's mad at me. There's nothing anybody can find out. A guilt-free conscience.

Verse 17. Be zealous. But be careful. Be zealous for the right things.

Verse 18. Keep your eye on the prize, not the momentary thrill. The fact of the matter is, sin is fun. If it wasn't fun, nobody would do it. But the problem is, the punishment for sin, the results of sin, last for years. Sometimes even a lifetime.

"Son, be wise, set your will, your heart on the right path." If you're going to act wisely, your heart has got to be set on the right things. But when we don't act righteously, that starts with our will. If you want to be righteous before God, it's a sacrifice of your will.

Verse 20, don't join those who drink too much wine or gorge themselves on meat. That's because an out of control style of life driven by something to feel, to medicate or fill a void, that is something other than God filling that void. You have a God shaped hole in your heart. Filling it with anything else, you will be sadly disappointed.

Drunkards and gluttons become poor. Drowsiness clothes them in rags. Folks who live like this, who live addicted to substance, whether it's food or alcohol or drugs, or themselves, they have difficulty becoming productive people because something else is in charge of their lives.

Look at what happens in Hollywood. These people have everything you would think you would ever want to live for and they find them dead in the gutter from an overdose. *Because something else is really in charge of their lives.* You and I would look at them and go, they've got it all! But the truth is somebody's got them. Something's got them.

And they end up destitute because *they're not in charge.*

"Listen to you father who gave you life…" [mama brought you in, mama can take you out] … "don't despise your mom when she's old.' But you should learn form her wisdom. Live a life of self-respect and honor your parents. Young people, the greatest thing you can do for your parents is listen. Just listen. If you choose to obey, good for you. If you choose not to obey, your day's coming. Because sooner or later, it all catches up to you. Right? You're better off listening to your parents because they survived being a teenager. They survived being a young adult. They survived being all that stuff. They might actually have something of value to say to you.

This is a great thing here for kids, for all of us. Buy the truth. Get wisdom. Don't sell the truth. The best thing you could ever get is the truth in your life. Nobody should be able to buy it from you. The price is too high, pal. I found Jesus, you're not cashing in on Jesus. I'm not giving up on this. Buy the truth. Don't sell it. Once you've got a hold of it, and it's got a hold on you, don't let go of it for just any old reason. Hold on to it.

"The father of a righteous child has great joy. The man who fathers a wise child rejoices in him. Of course. May your mother and father rejoice. May she who gave birth to you be joyful." Young people, the way you live matters because other people are watching. And it's a great deterrent that you don't want to do things that disappoint the people closest to you. You don't want to be a statistic.
"My son, give me your heart." Give me your will. Let your eyes delight in my ways. I want you to understand, the best thing parents can do is be an example because your kids will not always do what you say, but they will do what you do. And if they see you handle a certain circumstance in a certain way, that's probably how they're going to handle it. *You might have taught them otherwise, but they're almost always going to do what we do instead of do what we say.*

"An adulterous woman is a deep pit." [I guess an adulterous man is a deep pit too.] A wayward wife is a narrow well. Like a bandit, they wait, and lie, and multiply the unfaithful among them.'

Listen, sin's easy. And if you're lonely, you can go online or make a phone call. You'll find someone to pay attention to you. It might cost you a few dollars. But in the end, because you've sinned with your body, the only sin that is against your body, you'll pay for it. I'm not lying. I'm telling the truth.

When we do what our heart wants, something or someone who's now in the spot reserved for God, that thing steals your life from you. It steals your life from you. And in the end, the number of people that get hurt, you can't even being to imagine.

Verse 19 it kind of turns to the issue we would say of alcohol. "Who has woe? Who has sorrow? Who has strife? Who's complaining?" [Go ahead, the bartender's listening.] These guys should have degrees in counseling.

"Who has needless bruises and bloodshot eyes?" The guy who falls across the floor, that's who. He fell into the table. Nobody punched him.

"Don't gaze at the wine when it's red, when it sparkles in the cup." This had to do with the fermentation of grape juice. People could tell whether it was fermented by the way it sparkled just right.

"In the end it bites like a snake and poisons like a viper." Yeah, the morning after especially. It'll sit up and bite you if you've had too much.

"Your eyes will see strange sights. Your mind will imagine confusing things. You'll be like one on the high seas lying in the top of the rigging. Back and forth." We've all seen these people.

"They hit me!" No they didn't. "They hit me and I don't even feel it anymore. Where do I get another drink?" That's what it says.

I think you understand. It's a life of excess. And when we live a life that's based on excess and system overload, too much of anything, something, anything, that is gluttonous behavior.

Doesn't matter what it is. How much money is enough money? How many vacations are enough vacations? How much stuff is enough stuff? How much square feet is a big enough house? How new does the car have to be? How big does the engine have to be? When are you okay? *Because if the goal, if the pursuit, is always chasing something bigger and better, you've got to be careful because that becomes gluttonous behavior.*

Anything in my life, anything in your life, *that we cannot live without,* it's gluttony. Anything. We should be able to walk away from anything. Self-control, Spirit led. That's what the Bible teaches. *Anything that is in control of my life is something that's taken the place of God.* And if we're controlled by somebody, controlled by some circumstance, controlled by some substance, or controlled by some pursuit, that's where God belongs. It becomes gluttonous behavior on our part. Why? Because it's idolatrous. That's why.

"I am a jealous God. Punishing the children of the fathers." And later on in the Ten Commandments it says, "but showing love to a thousand generations of those who love me and keep my commandments." God isn't playing second base for anybody. He's not going to let you be in charge. He's not going to let me be in charge. He wants to be in charge. There's only one throne in your heart. You're on it. Or He's on it. And He's not going to stand and watch you sit on the throne.

What area of your life does gluttony affect you? What area? Because if you're reading this today and you don't have an issue, God bless you, please come see me. I want to know. At least I can be the only pastor in America that can say I have one person in my church that's not gluttonous. It's scary.

And it becomes so easy for us to look around and say, that person, that person, they do, he does, she does, and never look in the mirror at ourselves. Because it's really hard to stand there, facing yourself, and admit that guy does, that guy does, that guy does, when you're talking about yourself.

I can't change you. I can only change me. And as I told you in the last chapter, I can't change me, until I'm willing to submit to the Spirit and allow the Spirit to change me. And I'm asking you to be honest. What are you struggling with? Get over it. Allow God to minister to you and to take that off your plate.

Living Life On Purpose means living a life of Health: Spiritually, Mentally, Emotionally and Physically.

Commit yourself to this TODAY!

[Recipes Provided By Chef Kate Juneau, a Friends Community Church Family Member]

Chicken

Basil Chicken with Lemongrass Brown Rice and Green Bean Almondine
Yields 4 servings

4 Boneless, Skinless Chicken Breasts
8 Basil Leaves
1/4 C Extra Virgin Olive Oil
4 cloves Garlic; minced
2 stalks of Lemongrass
2 C Brown Rice
3 1/2 C Water
2 C Fresh Green Beans
3 T slivered Almonds
1 T Extra virgin olive oil
4 C water
1 T Lemon Juice
salt and pepper to taste

1. Place basil leaves, 2 cloves of minced garlic, the 1/4 C olive oil and a pinch of salt and pepper in a blender. Blend until smooth. Place chicken breasts in shallow bowl and cover with mixture. Let marinate in refrigerator for 2 hours.
2. Place chicken breasts on a sheet pan that has been sprayed with cooking spray [such as Pam]. Place in a 350 degree oven for 35 minutes or until chicken reaches an internal temperature of 160 degrees Fahrenheit.
3. Smash the stalks of lemongrass with a meat mallet or with the handle of a kitchen knife. Place in the 3 1/2 C of water and bring to a simmer. When the water is aromatic, remove the stalks and bring water to a boil. Add the rice, cover, reduce heat to a simmer and cook for approx. 20 minutes or until rice is done. (You can

also make it according to package directions after the lemongrass is steeped in the water.) Fluff with fork.

4. Bring 4 C of water to a boil. Blanch the green beans for 30 seconds and remove.
5. Place green beans in an ice bath.
6. Heat a skillet with the 1 T of olive oil to a medium heat. Add green beans, remaining garlic, a pinch of salt and pepper and saute'. Be careful not to burn the garlic. Place on a serving platter.
7. In the same skillet add the almonds and toss until toasted brown. Add the lemon juice and toss to coat. Pour over green beans.

Grilled Chicken with Herbed Red Bliss Potatoes and Steamed Veg Medley

Yields 4 servings

4 Boneless, skinless chicken breasts
2 T Italian seasoning with no MSG
2 lbs of red bliss potatoes
6 garlic cloves; smashed
1/2 lb of each cauliflower, broccoli, and baby carrots
2 T Extra virgin olive oil
salt, pepper, and granulated garlic to taste

1. Season chicken breasts with salt, pepper, and granulated garlic to taste. Place on grill and cook, turning only once, until an internal temperature of 160 degrees in reached.
2. Clean and quarter potatoes. Place in bowl with olive oil, Italian seasoning, smashed garlic, and a pinch of salt and pepper. Toss to coat. Place on a sheet pan in a single layer and bake at 350 degrees until golden brown. Approximately 40 minutes.
3. Fill a large pot with water just under a steaming basket (If you don't have one you can place a colander on top of the pan and it will work the same) Bring water to a boil and place veggies in either the steam basket or the colander and place a lid on top. Steam until vegetables are tender. Approximately 7-10 minutes.

Baked Chicken Fingers with Zucchini Fries and Cauliflower Mash

Yields 4 servings

4 Boneless, skinless chicken breasts; cut into thirds lengthwise
4 C of Panko breadcrumbs; divided
6 eggs, beaten; divided
2 medium sized zucchini
1 head of Cauliflower
2 T Butter
4 T Low fat plain greek yogurt
1/4 C Low fat cheese such as colby jack
2 t of Cayenne pepper
salt, pepper, and granulated garlic to taste

1. Season chicken tenders with salt, pepper, and granulated garlic to taste. Place 2 C of panko, and 3 beaten eggs in separate bowls. Take tenders, one by one, and dip in egg mixture then panko. Place on sheet tray and repeat until all tenders are finished. Bake at 350 until an internal temperature of 160 degrees is reached. Approximately 35 minutes.
2. Cut ends of zucchini, then cut in half; both lengthwise and width. Proceed to cut into sticks. Season with salt, pepper, and cayenne. Place remaining panko and eggs in separate bowls. Dip sticks in egg then panko. Place on sheet tray. Bake at 350 until golden brown. Approximately 30 minutes.
3. Cut the cauliflower into florets. Place in a pot with water and bring to a boil until tender. Drain. Return to pot with butter, Greek yogurt and a pinch of salt and pepper. Mash with a potato masher. You can adjust the consistency with more or less Greek yogurt. Top with cheese.

Whole Wheat Penne Pasta with Chicken and Garden Veggies

Yields 4 servings

4 boneless, skinless chicken breasts; cut into medium dice
1/2 lb Whole wheat penne pasta
1 small yellow onion; chopped
4 cloves of garlic; minced
1 28 oz can of diced tomatoes
1 bunch of Basil; chiffonade
1 C of sliced white mushrooms
2 C of fresh spinach
1 yellow Pepper; seeds removed and julienne
2 T Extra virgin olive oil; divided salt and pepper to taste

1. In Deep skillet over medium heat 1 T olive oil, yellow pepper, and chopped onion. Cook until onion is translucent then add chicken and garlic. Cook until chicken is brown. Add tomatoes and mushrooms. Simmer for 20 minutes. Add spinach and basil and cook until spinach is just wilted. Add salt and pepper to taste.
2. Bring a large pot of water to a boil. Add penne and cook until al dente. 7-9 minutes. Drain and toss with 1 T of olive oil.
3. Place penne in sauce and toss to coat.

Chicken Lettuce Wraps
Yields 4 servings

4 boneless, skinless chicken breasts, sliced thinly lengthwise
3 T low sodium Hoisin sauce
1 T low sodium soy sauce
1 T Fresh grated ginger
1 T Garlic; minced
3 Scallions, thinly sliced
3 heads of Boston baby bibb lettuce
3 medium carrots, peeled, and very thinly sliced
3 medium cucumbers, peeled, and very thinly sliced
1/4 C toasted almonds
Sweet chili sauce and/ or Ponzu for dipping

1. Combine chicken, hoisin, soy, ginger, garlic, and scallions in a bowl. Mix, cover and refrigerate for 2 hours.
2. Remove and wash leaves from lettuce. Set aside.
3. Drain off half of marinade and cook with chicken, in a saucepan, over medium heat until chicken is no longer pink.

4. Place a little carrot, cucumber, almonds, and chicken mixture in a baby bibb leaf. Roll up and dip in desired sauce.

Beef

Filet Mignon with Roasted Asparagus and Smashed Potatoes
Yields 4 servings

4- 4oz portions of center cut filet mignon.
1 bunch of Asparagus; ends trimmed
4T Extra Virgin Olive OIl
1 1/2 lbs of red bliss potatoes
salt, pepper, and granulated garlic to taste

1. Wash and quarter potatoes. Place in bowl with 2 T olive oil, salt, pepper, and granulated garlic to taste. Lay in a single layer on a sheet pan and bake for 25 minutes at 350 degrees. Take out of the oven and smash with a meat mallet or the back of a heavy pan. Place back in oven and bake for an additional 15 minutes.
2. Place trimmed asparagus in a saute' pan with 2 T of olive oil, and a pinch of salt and pepper. Saute' until Asparagus are brown and slightly wilted.
3. Season filet with salt and pepper. Grill, flipping only once, until an internal temperature of 145 degrees is reached.

Stuffed Peppers with Quinoa and Ground Beef
Yields 4 servings

2 C cooked Quinoa; prepared per package directions 1lb lean ground beef such as 80/20
4 big green peppers, tops removed and deseeded
1 16oz can of diced tomatoes with green chilies
4 cloves garlic; minced
1 small yellow onion; diced
2 T Tomato Paste
1 T Cumin
1 T Chili Powder
1 t Salt
1 t Pepper
1 C low fat shredded pepper jack cheese
1. Brown hamburger with garlic and onion over medium heat. Drain.
   2. Return hamburger to pan and add can of tomatoes, tomato paste, cumin, chili powder, salt, and pepper. Cook until heated through. Turn off heat and add quinoa. Mix until completely combined.
   3. Stuff mixture into green peppers. (Depending on the size of your peppers you may or may not have mixture remaining.)
   4. Place on a sheet pan and bake for 35 minutes in a 350 degree oven.
   5. Take out peppers, cover with cheese and bake another 10 minutes.

Asian Flank Steak with Scallion Rice and Roasted Peppers
Yields 4 servings

24 oz Flank Steak; trimmed
2 C Jasmine rice
3 1/2 C Water
6 Stalks scallions; thinly sliced and divided
4 T Extra Virgin Olive Oil; divided
1 Red bell pepper, cut julienne
1 Yellow bell pepper, cut julienne
1 Orange bell pepper, cut julienne
4 T Low sodium soy sauce
2 T Freshly grated ginger
2 T Garlic; minced
2 T Sesame Oil
2 T Lime zest
salt and pepper to taste

1. Combine soy sauce, ginger, garlic, sesame oil, lime zest and half of the scallions in a bowl. Mix. Pour over Flank steak and let rest while preparing the rice and peppers.
2. Prepare rice according to package directions or bring 3 1/2 C of water to a boil. Add rice, cover and reduce to a simmer. Cook 20 minutes or until rice has absorbed all of the water. Mix in 2 T of olive oil and scallions. Cover and keep warm.
3. Place julienne peppers in a bowl with 2 T of olive oil and salt and pepper to taste. Toss to coat. Spread on a sheet pan in a single layer and roast in the oven for 15-20 minutes at 350 degrees.
4. Grill flank steak, turning only once, until an internal temperature of 145 degrees is reached. Once off the grill, allow the meat to rest for 5-7 minutes. Slice thinly, against the grain, and on a bias for maximum tenderness.

Southwestern Burger with Black Bean Salsa and Chipotle Cream

Yields 4 servings

1-1 1/2 lb of lean ground beef, such as 80/20
1 10oz can of black beans, drained and rinsed
2 medium vine ripe tomato, deseeded and diced
1 small jalapeno', ribs and seeds removed, diced small
1 4oz can of corn, drained
1 lime, juiced
1 T Cumin
1 T Chili Powder
1 clove Garlic, minced
1 can of chipotle chiles in adobo sauce
4 oz of plain, low fat greek yogurt
4 whole wheat pitas, lightly toasted, cut in half to expose pocket
4 slices of low fat pepper jack cheese
1-2 C shredded lettuce
salt and pepper to taste

1. Combine beans, tomato, jalapeno', corn, lime juice, cumin, chili powder, garlic and a pinch of salt and pepper in a bowl. Set aside.
2. Combine Greek yogurt and sauce *only* from can of chipotles in small bowl. (reserve chipotle chiles for another use.) Add a pinch of salt and pepper. Set aside.
3. Make 4 4oz patties with ground beef. Grill, turning only once, until an internal temperature of 155 degrees is reached. Place a slice of cheese on right before pulling off the grill. It will melt with carry-over cooking time.
4. Stuff pita with lettuce, add the burger, salsa and chipotle cream.

Lean Beef Stew
Yields 4-6 servings

2 lbs of strip steak or stew meat, cut into cubes
1/4 C All purpose flour
1 t salt
1 t pepper
1 t cayenne pepper
6 cloves of garlic, smashed
2 bay leaves
1 t Worcestershire
1 medium yellow onion, chopped
3 russet potatoes; diced
4 carrots, peeled and chunked
2 stalks of celery; chunked
2 C low sodium beef broth
1/2 head of escarole, washed and cut into bite sized pieces
1. Place beef in crock pot. Mix the flour, salt, pepper, cayenne and pour over meat. Stir to coat. Add garlic, bay leaves, Worcestershire, onion, broth, potatoes, carrots, and celery. Cover and cook on low for 8-10 hours. Stir in escarole and cook until tender; approximately 20 minutes.

Fish

Blackened Tilapia with Mango Salsa and Cilantro Lime Rice
Yields 4 servings
4 Tilapia filets
2 T of Canola oil
1 Mango, peeled, seed removed and diced
1/4 of a pineapple, cleaned, cored, and diced
1 Red onion, diced
1 small red pepper, diced
2 limes, juiced and zest, divided
1 bunch of cilantro, chopped and divided
2 C Brown rice (Prepared according to package directions)
3 T of Blackening seasoning such as Paul Prudhomme's
Redfish Magic
Salt and pepper to taste

1. Combine diced mango, onion, pineapple, red pepper, the juice and zest of one lime, 1/4 C of cilantro, and salt and pepper in a bowl. Combine and set aside.
2. Prepare rice according to package directions. When finished, add the juice and zest of one lime and 1/2 C cilantro. Stir, cover, and keep warm.
3. Sprinkle tilapia filets with blackening seasoning.
4. Add 2 T oil to skillet and heat over medium heat. When the oil starts to smoke, add the filets seasoning side down. Cook for 3 minutes and flip. Cook an additional 2-3
   minutes or until center reaches 145 degrees.
5. Place rice in center of plate, and top with tilapia and mango salsa.

Mediterranean Salmon
Yields 4 servings

4 5oz Filets of wild caught salmon, cleaned and pin bones removed
2 C Spinach
1 28oz can of diced tomatoes
1/2 C Black olives, chopped
1/2 C Green olives, chopped
1/2 C Kalamata olives, chopped
1/4 C Capers
4 oz Extra Virgin Olive Oil
6 oz Feta Cheese
1 lemon, sliced
salt and pepper to taste
Tzatziki Sauce (Recipe Follows)
Tzatziki Sauce
16 oz of plain greek yogurt
2 cucumbers, peeled, seeded, and diced
1 T Extra virgin olive oil
1 lemon, juiced
2 T Fresh chopped dill
4 garlic cloves, minced
Salt and pepper to taste
Combine all ingredients *except yogurt* in a food processor until smooth. Fold in yogurt, then refrigerate. Process until well combined. Cover and refrigerate for one hour for best results.

1. Place diced tomatoes in the bottom of a square, 2" deep baking pan. Spread evenly on bottom of pan. Top with spinach making sure its even all over the pan. Place salmon filets on top. Season lightly with salt and pepper. Place lemon slices over fish.
2. Combine olives, capers, and 2 T of olive oil in food processor. Process until olives are all minced together. Place on top of salmon filets. Cover everything with Feta.

3. Cover with aluminum foil. Bake in a 350 degree oven for 40 minutes or until an internal thermometer reads 145 degrees.
4. Drizzle tzatziki sauce on top just before serving.

Baked Catfish with Sauteed Kale and Stuffed Tomatoes
Yields 4 servings

4 4-6oz catfish filets, cleaned and skinned removed
2 slices of low sodium bacon, thinly sliced
2 C of Kale, cut into bite sized strips
4 cloves of garlic, thinly sliced
2 T Olive oil
1/2 C Vegetable stock
2 T Red wine vinegar
1 C Cornmeal
2 eggs, beaten
4oz of garlic and herb goat cheese
4 Roma tomatoes, halved, and insides scooped out

1. Render bacon over low heat. When fully cooked and crispy, drain and reserve
2. Season catfish filets with salt and pepper. Dip into egg then cornmeal. Place on a sheet tray. Bake in a 350 degree oven for 40 minutes or until an internal thermometer reaches 145 degrees.
3. Spoon 1oz of goat cheese into tomato halves and spread evenly. Place on a sheet tray that has been sprayed with non stick coating. Bake for 25 minutes in a 350 degree oven.
4. Heat 2 T of olive oil in a saute' pan over medium heat. Add the garlic and cook until fragrant but not brown. Turn the heat up to medium high, add the stock and kale. Combine, cover and cook for 5 minutes. Remove the lid, continue to cook, stirring until all of the liquid has evaporated. Season with salt, pepper, and vinegar. Add bacon right before serving.

Fish Tacos
Yields 4 servings, 2 tacos per person

4 fish filets, a white fish such as tilapia or cod
2 T Canola oil
8 whole wheat tortillas
1/2 head of napa cabbage, shredded on a cheese grater
1/2 head of purple cabbage, shredded on a cheese grater
2 carrots, peeled and grated
juice and zest of 4 limes; divided
1/2 bunch of cilantro, chopped; divided
1 C plain Greek yogurt
2 cloves of garlic, minced

1. Season fish filets with salt and pepper.
2. Heat 2 T of oil in skillet. When it starts to smoke, add fish filets seasoned side down.
   Cook for 3 minutes and flip. Cook for an additional 2-3 minutes, or until an internal
   thermometer reaches 145 degrees.
3. In bowl, combine Napa cabbage, purple cabbage, carrots, juice and zest and juice of 2 limes, and salt and pepper to taste.
4. In separate bowl combine yogurt, juice and zest of 2 limes, chopped cilantro and salt and pepper to taste. Stir.
5. When fish filets are done, cut them in half lengthwise. Put some cabbage in a tortilla, put half a piece of fish on top, finish with cilantro cream.

Forbidden Rice with Shrimp, Peaches, and Snap Peas
Yields 4 servings

2 C Black Rice 3 1/2 C Water
2 T Fresh grated ginger
4 T olive oil, divided
1 1/2 lbs large shrimp, peeled and deveined
2 C Snap peas, cut into bite sized pieces
3 peaches, diced
1 T low sodium soy sauce
1 1/2 T rice wine vinegar
1 T Hoisin sauce

1. Prepare rice per package directions, but add a pinch of salt and the ginger to the pan you'll be cooking it in. When done, cover and keep warm.
2. In nonstick skillet, heat 1 T of oil over medium heat. Add shrimp and a pinch of both salt and pepper. Cook until opaque (4-6 minutes). Remove from pan.
3. In same pan, heat 1 T of oil. Add peas and peaches. Cook until warm but crisp.
4. In bowl mix remaining oil, soy sauce, hoisin sauce until smooth.
5. Place rice in bowl, top with shrimp, peas, and peaches. Finish with soy mixture.

FRUIT
Kebobs With Yogurt Dipping Sauce

1 pkg Strawberries, tops removed
1/2 of a Pineapple, cleaned, cored, chunked
1/2 of a Cantaloupe, cleaned, deseeded, chunked
1/2 of a Honey Dew, cleaned, deseeded, chunked
3 C Grapes, red or green seedless
2 C Plain Greek yogurt
1/4 C honey
1/4 C raspberries, smashed
1/4 C blackberries, smashed
1 pkg medium to long wooden kebob skewers
    1. Alternate fruit on kebob skewers.
    2. Combine yogurt sauce, honey, and smashed raspberries and blackberries in bowl. Stir well.
    3. Kebobs can be left as is or grilled.

Grilled Pineapple and Bananas
Yields 4 servings

1/2 Pineapple, cleaned, cored, and sliced into 1/2" slices
2 Bananas, cut in half lengthwise with skin on
Yields 8 servings

2 T Sugar in the raw
2 T ground cinnamon
4 T Honey
1/4 C toasted, unsweetened coconut
1 C Low fat vanilla ice cream
　1. Heat grill. (I do not recommend a George Foreman for this.)
　2. Drizzle pineapple and bananas with honey.
　3. Combine sugar and cinnamon and sprinkle on bananas only. Let them sit for 5 minutes.
　4. Place the pineapple and bananas (cut side DOWN) on the grill. Grill for 2 minutes then flip. Grill for 5 more minutes or until the skin pulls away from the bananas. Remove from grill and serve with 1/4 C low fat vanilla ice cream and a sprinkle of coconut.

Strawberry Fruit Leather
Yields 10 servings

1 pt of Strawberries
2 T honey

1. Place strawberries and honey in a blender or a food processor until it forms a paste.
2. Spread evenly on a baking sheet lined with parchment paper.
3. Bake in a 130 degree oven overnight or for 10 hours. Using the convection method on your oven will work best.
4. Cool before serving

Baked Apple Chips
Yields 10 servings

3 large Gala apples
2 T ground Cinnamon
> 1. Slice apples thinly. Cut out seeds on slices that apply.
> 2. Lay slices on parchment lined baking sheets. Sprinkle with cinnamon. Bake for 2 hours at 225 degrees, rotating the pan after 1 hour. Cool before serving

Applesauce
Yields 4 servings

3 lbs of peeled, cored, and chunked apples such as Fuji or Granny Smith
1/4 C Brown sugar
1/8 C Sugar in the Raw
1 C water
5 strips of lemon peel (Use vegetable peeler) 2 cinnamon sticks
Juice of 1/2 lemon
1. Put all ingredients in a medium pot. Cover and bring to boil. Lower heat and simmer for 25 minutes.
2. Remove from heat. Remove cinnamon sticks and lemon peel. Mash with potato masher or keep as is.
3. Ready to serve with low fat vanilla ice cream, low fat greek yogurt, pork tenderloin, or by itself.

Summer Treats

Watermelon Granita
Yields 8 servings

1/2 of a seedless watermelon, rind removed, and cut into chunks 2 limes, juiced
1/4 C Sugar

1. Place half of the watermelon, half the sugar, and half the lime juice in a blender. Blend until smooth and pour into a bowl. Repeat with other half of ingredients. Pour into same bowl of first mixture.
2. Pour entire mixture into a 9x13 baking dish. Place in the freezer for 2 hours.
3. Begin the process of lightly scraping the top. Use either a fork or spoon or alternate between layers. Place back in freezer for 2 hours. Take out and scrape again. Continue this pattern until the entire mixture is shaved.

Smoothies
Yields 4 servings

Your choice of 2-3 fruits. Any of these can be used fresh or frozen
4 -5 Strawberries
1 Banana
1/2 C Raspberries
1/2 C Blueberries
3/4 C Blackberries
1-2 Peaches
1 Mango
3/4 C Pineapple
Add in1-2 C of Cubed Ice
1/2 C Skim or Almond Milk or coconut water
1/2 C Plain lowfat yogurt

Optional:
1 C Spinach
1 T Flax seeds
1 T Protein powder [only if leading an active lifestyle]
1. Place 2-3 desired fruits, ice, desired liquid, yogurt and any optional ingredients in blender and blend until smooth.

Frozen Nibbles
Yields 12 servings

1 box vanilla wafer cookies
1/2 C Plain Greek yogurt
1/2 C Neufchatel cheese
Zest of 1 lemon
2 t honey
sliced berry of choice; raspberries, blueberries, blackberries, or strawberries mini cupcake pan and liners

> 1. Place mini cupcake liners in pan. Place a vanilla wafer cookie in each.
> 2. In mixer, with paddle attachment, combine yogurt, cheese, lemon zest and honey.
> 3. Place a spoonful on top of each wafer. Freeze for 3 hours.
> 4. Top with berries of choice.

Fruit Pops
Yields 12 servings

2 C Bananas
2 Mangos
2 T Agave Nectar
Store bought popsicle mold
1. Blend bananas, mangos, and agave nectar in blender, or pulse several times for a chunkier popsicle.
2. Pour into molds. Leave the top off.
3. Freezer for one hour, place tops on.
4. Freeze 3 additional hours.

You can use any combinations of fruit for these popsicles.

Snacks

Peanut Butter and Apples
Yields 1 serving

1 apple of your choosing
2 T peanut butter
1 T Honey
1 slice of whole grain bread
> 1. Core and slice apples.
> 2. Toast bread, spread on Peanut butter and drizzle honey.

You can forego the toast, mix the honey and peanut butter to dip your apples in.

Caprese Skewers
Yields 8 servings

1 pt of Grape Tomatoes
16 pieces of Ciligene Mozzarella
Balsamic glaze
Frill toothpicks or small wooden skewers
> 1. Alternate pieces of tomato and Mozz on Skewers with a tomato, a mozz, then a tomato. 3 pieces total per skewer. Continue until all product is used.
> 2. Place on serving tray and drizzle with balsamic glaze.

Hard Cooked Eggs with Ants on a Log
Yields 1 serving

2 eggs
1 stalk celery, washed
8-10 raisins
2 T Peanut Butter

1. Place 2 eggs in a medium sauce pan and cover with cold water.
2. Place on stove and bring to a rolling boil. As soon as the eggs reach a rolling boil,
   take the pan off the heat, cover it, and let sit for 28 minutes. (This can be done up to 3
   days in advance)
3. Peel eggs.
4. Spread peanut butter in groove of celery stalk. Top with Raisins.

Trail Mix
Yields 8 servings

1/2 C Unsalted Peanuts
1/2 C Unsalted Almonds
1/2 C Unsalted Cashews
1/2 C Craisins
1/2 C Banana chips
!/2 C Dried Pineapple
1/2 C Dried Apricots
!/2 C Dried Mango
1/2 C Cheerios
1/4 C Unsalted Sunflower Seeds 1/4 C Hemp Seeds
1/2 C Plain Chex cereal
1/4 C Dark Chocolate chips
1/4 C Mini Marshmallows
1/2 C Air popped popcorn

1. Create your own combination. Make sure to keep it balanced. Stay away from dried fruits high in sugar.

Hummus
Yields 8 servings

1- 16 oz can of chickpeas, drained and rinsed
4 cloves of garlic, minced
1 T of Tahini sauce
1 T of Extra Virgin Olive Oil
1/2 T of Sesame Oil
Juice of 1 Lemon
salt, pepper, and Cayenne to taste
Baby Carrots
4 Celery stalks, cut into 1/4ths Pita bread, toasted

1. In the mixer with the paddle attachment, or in a food processor combine chickpeas, garlic, tahini, oils, juice of lemon, salt, pepper, and cayenne. Mix until completely combined, and smooth with a few chunks for texture.
2. Pour in bowl and serve with carrots, celery, or toasted pita bread.

Resources from

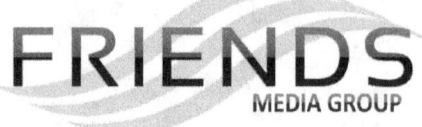

FRIENDS
MEDIA GROUP

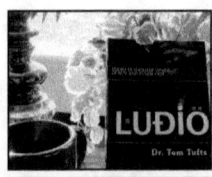

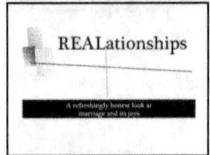

LUDIO: Leadership Upside Down and Inside Out
Study Guide/Small Group Discussion Book
Everyone is a leader! Leadership is most effective when it is done by seving people! And it's the most *fun* when you are leading from the heart!
Paperback or E-Book $9.99

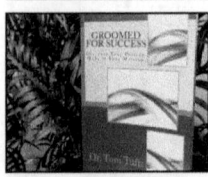

REALationships: A Refreshingly Honest Look at Marriage
and It's Joys
Rediscover *why* you got married and how to make it last! This is an in-depth, powerful series for individual couples and small group study.
6 week Workbook/Small Group Discussion Format
Paperback or E-book $9.99

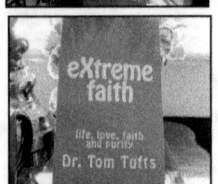

Groomed For Success: Find Your Passion; Make it Your Mission

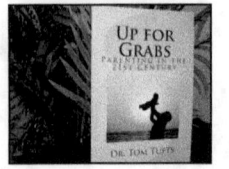

What are the traits that make people a success? Find out how communication, perspiration, delegation and participation will take you on a journey toward personal fulfillment! Paperback and e-book $7.99

eXtreme faith: life, love, faith and purity
Discover what it means to be a follower of Christ who lives a life of faith to the eXtreme! Easy to read, great stories and eXamples to impact your life!
Paperback and e-book $7.99

Up for Grabs: Parenting in the 21st Century
Times, they are 'a changing' as they say! Learn some simple principles and processes that can help you with your children. This book will help you understand *why they do what they do* and how you can help them become balanced, well-adjusted children. And you will be balanced, too! Paperback and e-book $7.99

Love You Love Notes
For Couples #1-100 To Her #1-100 To Him #1-100 To Kids #1-100
www.loveyoulovenotes.com

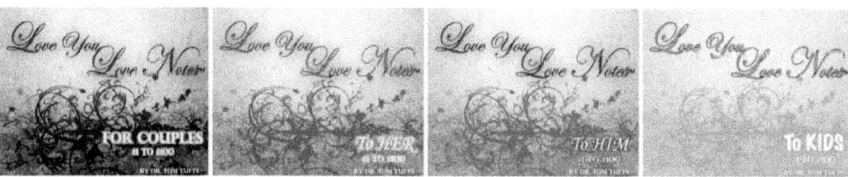

Also Check Out:

For scheduling information for Dr. Tom Tufts
www.tomtufts.com

For Additional Products:
　　　Shirts, Hats, Gear, Music CDs, Videos, Books, and more
　　　www.friendsmediagroup.com

Cover Designs:　　　In Demand Speakers, Orlando, FL
　　　www.indemandspeakers.com

www.ingramcontent.com/pod-product-compliance
Lightning Source LLC
Chambersburg PA
CBHW060405290526
45791CB00002B/621